# Clinical Nutrition
# the Dog and Cat

CW00408482

# LIBRARY OF VETERINARY PRACTICE

LIBRARY OF VETERINARY PRACTICE

# Clinical Nutrition of the Dog and Cat

**J.W. SIMPSON**
SDA, BVM&S, MPhil, MRCVS
Senior Lecturer
Royal (Dick) School of Veterinary Studies
Edinburgh

**R.S. ANDERSON**
BVMS, PhD, MRCVS
Professor of Animal Husbandry
University of Liverpool

**P.J. MARKWELL**
BSc, BVetMed, MRCVS
Waltham Centre for Pet Nutrition
Melton Mowbray

OXFORD

BLACKWELL SCIENTIFIC PUBLICATIONS

LONDON EDINBURGH BOSTON

MELBOURNE PARIS BERLIN VIENNA

© 1993 by
Blackwell Scientific Publications
Editorial Offices:
Osney Mead, Oxford OX2 0EL
25 John Street, London WC1N 2BL
23 Ainslie Place, Edinburgh EH3 6AJ
238 Main Street, Cambridge
  Massachusetts 02142, USA
54 University Street, Carlton
  Victoria 3053, Australia

Other Editorial Offices:
Librairie Arnette SA
2, rue Casimir-Delavigne
75006 Paris
France

Blackwell Wissenschafts-Verlag
Meinekestrasse 4
D-1000 Berlin 15
Germany

Blackwell MZV
Feldgasse 13
A-1238 Wien
Austria

First published 1993

Set by Excel Typesetters Company,
Hong Kong
Printed and bound in Great Britain
at the Alden Press, Oxford

DISTRIBUTORS

Marston Book Services Ltd
PO Box 87
Oxford OX2 0DT
(*Orders*: Tel: 0865 791155
      Fax: 0865 791927
      Telex: 837515)

USA
Blackwell Scientific Publications, Inc.
238 Main Street
Cambridge, MA 02142
(*Orders*: Tel: 800 759-6102
        617 876-7000)

Canada
Times Mirror Professional Publishing, Ltd
130 Flaska Drive
Markham, Ontario L6G 1B8
(*Orders*: Tel: 800 268-4178
        416 470-6739)

Australia
Blackwell Scientific Publications Pty Ltd
54 University Street
Carlton, Victoria 3053
(*Orders*: Tel: 03 347-5552)

A catalogue record for this title
is available from the British Library

ISBN 0-632-03363-0

Library of Congress
Cataloging-in-Publication Data

Simpson, J.W.
    Clinical nutrition of the dog and cat/
J.W. Simpson, R.S. Anderson,
P.J. Markwell.
      p.      cm.
    (Library of veterinary practice)
    Includes bibliographical references
and index.
    ISBN 0-632-03363-0
    1. Dogs—Diseases—Nutritional aspects.
    2. Cats—Diseases—Nutritional aspects.
    3. Nutrition disorders in animals.
    4. Dogs—Nutrition.   5. Cats—Nutrition.
    I. Anderson, Ronald S. (Ronald Shand).
    II. Markwell, P.J.   III. Title.   IV. Series.
SF992.N88S56   1993
636.7′0895854—dc20

# Contents

# Preface

Considering the number of dogs and cats in the United Kingdom it is surprising that relatively few textbooks exist on the subject of small animal nutrition. The majority of textbooks concentrate on the farm animal species, where a sound knowledge of nutrition has always been economically important. Farmers and veterinary surgeons have developed systems of nutritional management which have resulted in better health and improved productivity.

It is only recently that the importance of dog and cat nutrition has been established. In particular, the production of a wide range of veterinary diets has provided the small animal clinician with an important therapeutic tool to assist in the management of systemic diseases. Clients have also become more nutritionally aware and interested in the role of diet in the health of their pet.

The nutritional management of clinical disease is becoming part of everyday small animal practice and there is an increasing demand for more information on this subject.

The purpose of this book is to provide the practitioner, undergraduate and veterinary nurse with a practical guide to nutrition in the dog and cat. It is not a definitive text but an introduction to clinical nutrition and we hope the reader will find that nutrition can be an interesting and exciting subject with many opportunities to provide better health for the pets in their care. If we achieve this we will be more than satisfied.

# Acknowledgements

Table 1.1 and Figs 1.3, 1.4, 1.6, 1.7 and 1.9–1.13 are reproduced, with permission, from *Digestive Disease in the Dog and Cat* (Blackwell Scientific Publications, Oxford). Table 2.3 is produced with permission from the National Academy Press, and Table 2.4 with permission from Macmillan Magazines Ltd and the British Veterinary Association. We would also like to take this opportunity to thank Mr A.G. Burnie for providing Figs 3.2–3.4, Mr A.D.H. van den Broek for providing Fig. 3.5, and Mr J. Evans MRCVS of Henston Ltd for permission to use the table of body weights for different breeds of dog shown as Appendix 1.

# 1 / Anatomy and Physiology of the Digestive Tract

## Introduction

Before the nutritional requirements of the dog and cat can be met, ingested food must be digested and absorbed from the digestive tract. A knowledge of these functions is essential in order to understand how the major food components are utilized by the dog and cat. The intention of this chapter is not to provide a definitive description of the digestive tract, but to summarize its functional anatomy and physiology. The emphasis has been placed on the important aspects of digestion and absorption, and how malnutrition can develop when these processes fail.

The digestive tract may be described as a hollow tube which starts at the mouth and terminates at the anus. Along its length various modifications take place to allow ingested nutrients to be processed and utilized.

The inner surface of the digestive tract, termed the mucosa (a mucous membrane), is composed of epithelial cells and mucus-secreting goblet cells. Modifications of the mucosa occur at various locations, such as the stomach and intestine, in order to carry out specific functions. The remaining structure of the gut wall is similar throughout the digestive tract. The sub-mucosal layer lies immediately under the mucosa and is rich in blood vessels and nerves. This is surrounded by smooth muscle composed of an inner circular and outer longitudinal layer. The whole gut is enclosed in a thin sheet of epithelial cells called the serosa (Evans & Christensen, 1979) (Fig. 1.1). At specific locations the circular muscle fibres become thickened forming sphincters which act like gates and control the movement of ingesta along the digestive tract.

The muscle fibres of the digestive tract produce two different types of contraction termed segmented and peristaltic contractions (Fig. 1.2).

Segmentation is the primary type of contraction associated with the digestive tract and involves alternate contraction and relaxation of neighbouring segments of the intestine. The purpose of this is to ensure thorough mixing of the intestinal contents to improve the efficiency of digestion and absorption. Segmentation is not associated with movement of ingesta along the intestine.

Peristalsis involves contraction of the muscle fibres behind a bolus of food together with relaxation of the muscle fibres immediately in front of it. This type of contraction does not mix the ingesta but is designed for transporting it from one part of the digestive tract to another.

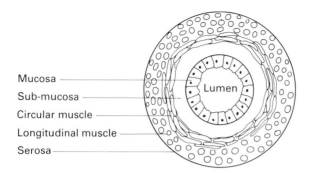

Mucosa

Sub-mucosa

Circular muscle

Longitudinal muscle

Serosa

**Fig. 1.1** Transverse section through the digestive tube showing the various layers of tissue present.

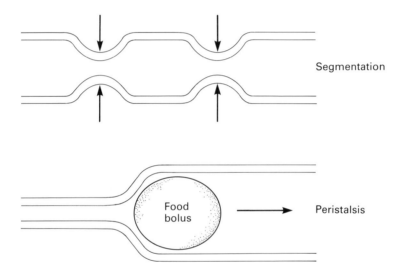

Segmentation

Food bolus

Peristalsis

**Fig. 1.2** The two forms of intestinal motility observed in the dog and cat.

The digestive tract may be divided into the following regions: the oral cavity, pharynx, oesophagus, stomach, small intestine, large intestine, rectum and anus. The pancreas and liver are important organs associated with the digestive tract.

## Oral cavity

The oral cavity is enclosed within the lips, cheeks, hard palate and tongue. The entire surface is covered by mucous membrane except for the crowns of the teeth. The lips and cheeks are designed to assist in the retention of food within the mouth. The tongue has several functions which include:

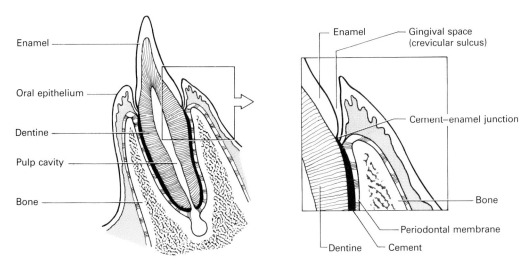

**Fig. 1.3** Structure of the tooth and peridonium. (From Simpson & Else, 1991.)

participating in the swallowing process, formation of a 'ladle' to permit drinking and the provision of taste buds.

The teeth in dogs and cats are designed for biting, tearing and shearing food rather than chewing. Consequently food is often swallowed in chunks which are then homogenized by the gastric contractions. The teeth are composed of an outer enamel layer which surrounds the dentine and inner pulp cavity (Fig. 1.3). Incisors, canines, premolars and molars are present. The fourth upper premolar and first lower molar teeth are also known as the carnassial teeth, and are designed for shearing meat. Both dogs and cats are born with deciduous teeth which are replaced by a permanent dentition from 4 months of age. The dental formulae of the two species are different (Table 1.1).

Several paired salivary glands (compound tubuloacinar glands) have ducts which drain directly into the oral cavity. The names of the salivary

**Table 1.1** The dental formulae in dogs and cats. (From Simpson & Else, 1991.)

|  | Dog | Cat |
|---|---|---|
| Deciduous | 3I  1C  3M | 3I  1C  3M |
|  | 3I  1C  3M | 3I  1C  2M |
| Permanent | 3I  1C  4PM  2M | 3I  1C  3PM  1M |
|  | 3I  1C  4PM  3M | 3I  1C  3PM  1M |

C − canine, I = incisor, M = molar, PM − premolar.

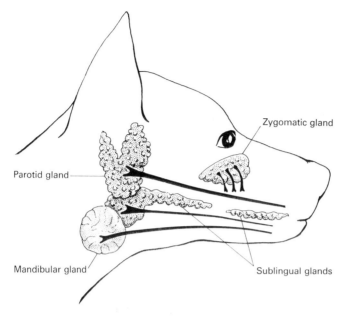

**Fig. 1.4** Location of the salivary glands and their ducts in the dog. (From Simpson & Else, 1991.)

glands relate to their locations and include the parotid, mandibular, sub-lingual and zygomatic glands (Fig. 1.4). The secretion produced by the salivary glands is alkaline, rich in bicarbonate, but contains no enzymes. There is no evidence that saliva carries out any enzymatic digestion (Simpson *et al.*, 1984) and the primary role in the dog and cat is lubrication of food. Failure to produce saliva results in difficulty in swallowing and food may be retained in the pharynx or oesophagus.

## Pharynx

The pharynx is a complex structure which forms a communication between the oral cavity, oesophagus, nasal passages and the lungs. The following six structures open into the pharynx: the oropharynx, the nasopharynx, two Eustachian tubes, the trachea and the oesophagus (Fig. 1.5). Like the other parts of the digestive tract, the pharynx is covered by mucous membrane, and has powerful muscles in its lateral walls.

## Oesophagus

The oesophagus is a simple muscular tube which transports food from the pharynx to the stomach. The muscle layer is highly developed and is almost entirely composed of skeletal muscle in the dog, while the caudal third of

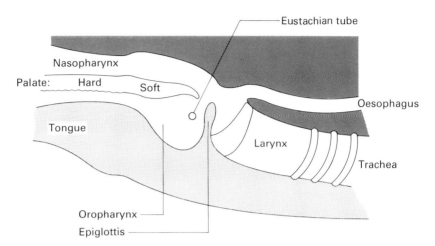

**Fig. 1.5** Anatomical arrangement of the pharynx, which is important with regard to the swallowing process.

the oesophagus contains smooth muscle in the cat. The cricopharyngeal sphincter at the cranial end of the oesophagus permits food to enter from the pharynx. At the distal end of the oesophagus there is no true sphincter, but a high pressure zone called the cardia helps to reduce the reflux of gastric contents. When empty the oesophagus is a collapsed tube with longitudinal folds. The caudal oesophagus in cats has a herring-bone appearance due to elastic fibres which result in pronounced mucosal folding. The mucosa contains many goblet cells which secrete large amount of mucus to assist in the lubrication of food during swallowing.

## Swallowing

Swallowing (deglutition) is a complex process which relies on intact sensory and motor innervation supplied by several of the cranial nerves. The process of swallowing is divided into three stages. The first stage is voluntary while the latter two stages are involuntary. Problems with swallowing are not uncommon and are usually due to defective innervation resulting in incoordination of the swallowing process. When this occurs the animal may lose a considerable amount of weight due to an inability to ingest an adequate quantity of food and may often inhale food giving rise to aspiration pneumonia.

Swallowing is initiated by the formation of a food bolus within the mouth. This is pushed against the hard palate by the tongue and then projected caudally into the pharynx. Sensory receptors in the pharynx initiate the second stage of swallowing by detecting the bolus, and reflexly closing the nasopharynx by upward movement of the soft palate, closing the

Eustachian tubes and sealing the larynx with the epiglottis. The pharyngeal muscles contract while the cricopharyngeal sphincter relaxes, forcing the bolus of food into the oesophagus. The last stage involves detection of the food bolus in the cranial oesophagus. This produces a primary peristaltic contraction moving the bolus down the oesophagus into the stomach. A second peristaltic wave often occurs which ensures the oesophagus has been completely emptied of food.

One of the commonest causes of difficulty in swallowing is mega-oesophagus. In this condition the oesophagus fails to contract; food is trapped in the oesophagus from whence it is eventually regurgitated and sometimes inhaled. The resulting inability to obtain adequate nutrition together with aspiration pneumonia usually result in weight loss and respiratory difficulty.

## Stomach

The stomach is a direct continuation of the oesophagus, acting as a reservoir for ingested food and initiating the process of digestion. It is divided into different zones (Fig. 1.6); the cardia is a small area associated with the oesophageal opening into the stomach, while the fundus acts as the reservoir

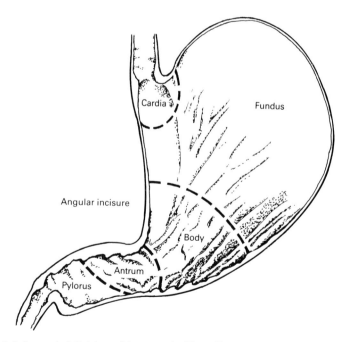

**Fig. 1.6** Anatomical divisions of the stomach. (From Simpson & Else, 1991.)

for ingested food. The antrum and pylorus function as the gastric grinder responsible for homogenizing ingested food into chyme. Gastric contents are released in a controlled manner through the pylorus, into the duodenum.

When the stomach is empty the fundal mucosa is thrown into folds called rugae due to the action of elastic and muscle fibres. The rugae disappear as the stomach fills with food. The gastric mucosa is composed of columnar epithelial cells and goblet cells which are renewed from germinal centres in the gastric pits. Goblet cells are found in the cardia, while specialised glands within gastric pits are found throughout the fundus and body of the stomach. Parietal cells in the mid-region of the gastric pits secrete hydrochloric acid while chief cells found near the base of the pits secrete pepsinogen, an inactive protease enzyme.

The gastric mucosal barrier is designed to protect the stomach from ingested irritants, hydrochloric acid and pepsin. The barrier is formed from a layer of mucus covering the epithelial cells, the epithelial cells themselves and the rich vascular bed in the submucosa. In addition to the physical barrier created by the epithelial cells, the mucus contains a phospholipid with hydrophobic properties in addition to pepsin inhibitors and has some buffering capacity against hydrochloric acid. Damage to this barrier results in inflammation (gastritis) and eventually ulceration. Eating becomes painful and the animal may vomit after eating or become anorexic resulting in weight loss.

When food is ingested the fundus usually relaxes to accommodate the meal without an increase in intragastric pressure; this is called receptive relaxation. If the stomach is inflamed or gastric motility is disturbed receptive relaxation does not occur and intragastric pressure rapidly increases leading to vomition associated with feeding.

The sight, smell and taste of food, together with the presence of food in the stomach, stimulate the secretion of hydrochloric acid and pepsinogen. Gastrin, a hormone produced by the stomach and intestine, also stimulates acid secretion together with antral contractions (Walsh *et al.*, 1972). Pepsinogen is converted to active pepsin by the presence of hydrochloric acid but is rapidly inactivated if the pH rises, which happens naturally when gastric contents enter the duodenum, where pancreatic bicarbonate neutralizes gastric acid. Both hydrochloric acid and pepsin initiate the process of digestion by hydrolysing proteins and starch.

The stomach has an inbuilt pacemaker located in the greater curvature which produces five slow waves per minute, some of which initiate muscle contractions (Weber & Kohatsu, 1970). Three types of gastric motility are recognized: digestive, intermediate and interdigestive patterns.

The digestive motility pattern is observed after ingestion of a meal. It involves a slow steady contraction of the fundus which supplies food to the antral grinder and empties liquids through the pylorus. The powerful peristaltic contractions of the antrum against a closed pylorus rapidly grind solid food to a small particle size (2 mm) which is then permitted to empty into the duodenum. When the meal is finished a transitional period of diminished gastric contractions occurs giving rise to the intermediate motility pattern. During periods when the stomach is empty interdigestive contractions occur, which involve sweeping peristaltic contractions of the whole stomach, emptying any contents into the duodenum. These are often termed 'housekeeper contractions' (Simpson & Else, 1991).

Following antral grinding of solid food the chyme produced is emptied into the duodenum in an orderly manner. Liquids empty before chyme, while proteins and carbohydrates empty before fats; undigestible material is last to leave the stomach. Meals rich in calories reduce the rate of gastric emptying; conversely meals with low calorie density empty more rapidly (Hunt & Stubbs, 1975). In this way, the stomach ensures the small intestine is never overwhelmed with chyme which would prevent efficient digestion and absorption from taking place. Where gastric motility disorders occur, disorganized emptying may lead to chyme flooding the small intestine, and inadequate digestion and absorption results in osmotic diarrhoea. Other signs associated with gastric motility disorders are the retention of food in the stomach for protracted periods of time and vomit associated with feeding.

In acute gastritis it is usual to withold food until vomiting stops. The acute inflammation is associated with disordered gastric motility which is manifest as gastric stasis and increased intragastric pressure when food is ingested. Both these situations result in vomition of the ingested food. In addition the physical presence of food on the inflamed mucosa causes irritation and leads to reflex vomiting.

Once vomiting subsides it is usual to offer a bland diet containing highly digestible ingredients which are low in fat, in several small meals daily. This routine serves several important purposes. Firstly highly digestible foods move rapidly through the stomach; a process which is accelerated by the use of food low in fat. This reduces the time food is retained in the stomach and so reduces any irritation to the mucosa and gastric stasis. Feeding several small meals during the day ensures the stomach is never full and so reduces the risk of increasing intragastric pressure and so recurrence of vomiting. Food which tends to be more abrasive such as dry biscuit should also be avoided at this time as it tends to irritate the healing gastric mucosa. For this reason moist foods are usually preferred.

If such a dietary regime is successful with no recurrence of vomiting, a slow return to the normal diet may proceed over a period of several days. There is a common tendency to carry out this stage too rapidly resulting in a relapse due to gastric irritation and increased intragastric pressure.

## Small intestine

The small intestine commences at the pylorus and terminates at the ileo-caecocolic junction. It is divided into three parts: the duodenum, jejunum and ileum. The duodenum is the first and shortest section of small intestine and is the site where the pancreatic and bile ducts enter the intestine. The jejunum and ileum form the main part of the small intestine and are suspended from the dorsal wall of the abdomen on a long mesentery permitting the intestine to form coils. There is no clear demarcation between the different parts of the small intestine.

The intestinal wall contains the same layers as the other parts of the digestive tract, although the mucosa has become specialized in order to carry out the main functions of the small intestine, namely the digestion and absorption of food. The epithelial cells lining the small intestine are called enterocytes and the whole mucosa is thrown up into folds called villi. On the apical surface of each enterocyte are finger-like processes called microvilli often termed the brush border (Simpson & Else, 1991) (Fig. 1.7). The formation of villi and microvilli significantly increases the surface area of the small intestine.

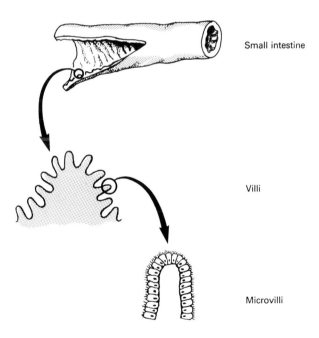

Small intestine

Villi

Microvilli

**Fig. 1.7** The formation of villi and microvilli in the small intestine, providing a large surface area for absorption. (From Simpson & Else, 1991.)

The crypts of Lieberkühn lie at the base of the villi and are the site for enterocyte renewal. It is here that the ducts of the tubuloalveolar glands empty their secretion into the crypts. The new enterocytes produced in the crypts of Lieberkühn migrate slowly up the villi to the tips where they are eventually shed into the lumen. This is a continual process which is completed every 4 days (Eastwood, 1977). The enterocytes mature as they migrate up the villi, so the cells with the greatest digestive and absorptive capacity are found at the tips. This has important practical significance because many viral infections damage the tips of the villi, resulting in marked loss of digestive and absorptive capacity. Goblet cells are found between the enterocytes and are responsible for secreting protective mucus. Endocrine cells are also found in the mucosa and are responsible for producing hormones which stimulate pancreatic and biliary secretions.

Each villus contains a rich vascular bed and a single blind-ended lymphatic vessel called a lacteal (Fig. 1.8). These vessels are responsible for the transport of absorbed nutrients from the small intestine to the liver and other body tissues.

The majority of the digestion and absorption of food is carried out in the small intestine and this is achieved in four ways:

**1** Intraluminal digestion involving the production of enzymes from the stomach and exocrine pancreas as well as bile salts.

**2** Mechanical digestion brought about by segmented contractions.

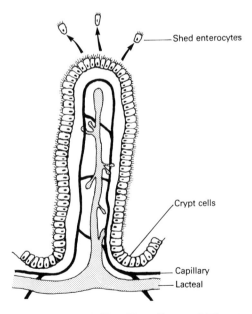

Shed enterocytes

Crypt cells

Capillary

Lacteal

**Fig. 1.8** Structure of the small intestinal villus. (From Simpson & Else, 1991.)

3   Mucosal digestion involving enzymes attached to the microvilli of the enterocytes which completes the process of digestion initiated in the lumen.
4   The absorption of end products of digestion into the enterocytes followed by their movement into the capillaries or lacteals.

The duodenum is relatively porous and has the capacity to secrete large volumes of fluid into the lumen which ensures the chyme from the stomach is kept isotonic. This degree of permeability progressively diminishes in the jejunum, ileum and colon so that only resorption of fluid can take place. In this way body fluids are conserved and diarrhoea is prevented.

The sight, smell and taste of food stimulates secretion of exocrine pancreatic enzymes and discharges of bile from the gall bladder. Hormonal stimulation is also important and occurs in response to the presence of acid chyme and nutrients in the duodenum. The production of cholecystokinin from the intestinal mucosa is stimulated by the presence of amino acids and fats; it stimulates the production of a pancreatic secretion rich in enzymes and causes contraction of the gall bladder. Secretin, also produced from the intestinal mucosa in response to acid chyme, produces a pancreatic secretion rich in bicarbonate and low in enzymes.

**Protein digestion**

Protein digestion is initiated in the stomach by the action of pepsin and hydrochloric acid. However the majority of protein digestion occurs in the small intestine (Argenzio, 1980). Inactive protease enzymes from the exocrine pancreas are secreted into the duodenum where enterokinase from the duodenal mucosa converts trypsinogen into active trypsin. Once activated trypsin is able to activate more of itself and the other protease enzymes, including chymotrypsin, carboxypeptidase and elastase.

Trypsin, chymotrypsin and elastase split proteins into smaller peptide chains, while carboxypeptidases A and B cleave the terminal amino acids from peptides liberating free amino acids. Nucleic acids are split by ribonuclease and deoxyribonuclease (Fig. 1.9).

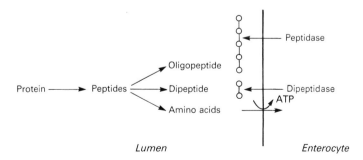

**Fig. 1.9** The process of protein digestion in the small intestine. (From Simpson & Else, 1991.)

Free amino acids are presented to the brush border for absorption. The dipeptides are too large for immediate absorption and are subjected to further digestion by a series of peptidase enzymes located on the brush border (Tobey *et al.*, 1985) (Fig. 1.9). Amino acids are absorbed into the enterocytes on specific carriers by an energy-dependent active process. Different carriers are used for different classes of amino acids. Once absorbed into the enterocytes the amino acids are liberated into the capillary bed of the villi and transported to the liver via the portal vein. Small amounts of amino acids are retained to assist in normal enterocyte function.

**Carbohydrate digestion**

The majority of carbohydrate consumed by adult dogs and cats is in the form of starch, although small amounts of simple sugars such as lactose and sucrose may also be ingested. Other forms of carbohydrate such as cellulose and hemicellulose, major types of dietary fibre, cannot be digested because suitable enzymes are not present in the digestive tract of the dog and cat.

Starch is composed of amylose and amylopectin. The amylose consists of linear chains of glucose units joined by $\alpha$ 1–4 bonds while amylopectin is composed of branched chains of glucose units joined by $\alpha$ 1–4 and $\alpha$ 1–6 bonds (Fig. 1.10). Digestion of starch in the small intestine is carried out by pancreatic $\alpha$ amylase which splits $\alpha$ 1–4 bonds but not $\alpha$ 1–6 bonds. The products of this digestion include small amounts of glucose together with maltose, maltotriose and limited dextrins (McDonald *et al.*, 1988) (Fig. 1.11).

The majority of products of starch digestion are too large to be absorbed by the enterocyte and must undergo further digestion on the brush border by disaccharidase enzymes including; lactase, sucrase, maltase and isomaltase. These enzymes are responsible for hydrolysis of lactose in milk, sucrose in sugar and products of starch digestion, yielding glucose and smaller amounts of fructose and galactose. Specific carriers on the enterocytes absorb these monosaccharides by an active energy-requiring process, against a concentration gradient (Tennant & Hornbuckle, 1980). Once in the

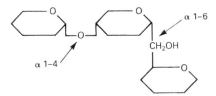

**Fig. 1.10** The method of linkage between glucose units in the starch molecule. (From Simpson & Else, 1991.)

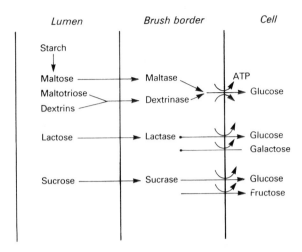

**Fig. 1.11** The process of carbohydrate digestion in the small intestine. (From Simpson & Else, 1991.)

enterocytes glucose is rapidly released into the capillaries and transported to the liver via the portal vein. The rapid movement of glucose into the capillaries assists in reducing the concentration gradient between the lumen and enterocytes.

## Fat digestion

Dietary fat is mainly composed of triglyceride which is very efficiently digested and absorbed. Other forms of fat may also be ingested including cholesterol and phospholipid, but they are less efficiently digested. The majority of triglyceride in the diet contains fatty acids with more than 12 carbon atoms which are termed long chain triglycerides (LCT). Triglycerides with between 8 and 12 carbon atoms are termed medium chain triglycerides (MCT) and those with less than 8 carbon atoms in the fatty acid chain are called short chain triglycerides (SCT) (Simpson & Doxey, 1983). An understanding of these different types of triglyceride is important when the digestion and absorption of dietary fat is considered.

Digestion of LCT starts in the small intestine by the action of lipase and bile salts (Fig. 1.12). As the luminal contents are aqueous, bile salts are essential for the production of a lipid/water interface to permit lipase digestion of the triglyceride. Without this detergent action no digestion of fat could occur even if large amounts of lipase were present. Segmented intestinal contractions ensure thorough mixing of the fat, lipase and bile salts, forming an emulsion of small fat droplets called micelles. This increases the water solubility of the fat and increases the surface area of fat for digestion, ensuring maximum lipase activity. The products of lipase

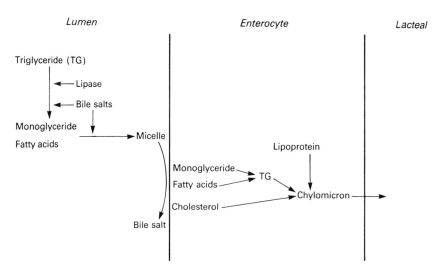

**Fig. 1.12** The process of fat digestion in the small intestine. (From Simpson & Else, 1991.)

digestion are monoglyceride and two free fatty acids. They are transported to the brush border in the micelle where they are absorbed passively into the enterocytes (Fig. 1.12). As the enterocyte cell membrane is lipid the process of absorption can occur passively and often occurs in association with absorption of fat soluble vitamins.

Within the enterocyte the fatty acids reform into triglyceride and attach to lipoproteins to form chylomicrons. The chylomicrons are released into the lacteal for transportation to the general circulation and subsequently to the liver and other tissues.

MCT and SCT are more water soluble and require less bile salt activity for lipase digestion. Absorption may also occur without the need for micelle formation. Although lipase digestion of these fats does occur, they may both be absorbed intact into enterocytes without any prior digestion. Chylomicrons are not formed in the enterocyte and the MCT and SCT are released directly into the capillaries and transported to the liver via the portal vein. This is why MCT is considered a useful source of calories in animals with malabsorption, especially lymphangectasia where the lymphatic circulation from the intestine becomes non-functional.

During a large meal there is an inadequate bile salt pool, and for this reason bile salts are conserved. Following fat digestion and absorption, bile salts are resorbed from the ileum and are transported to the liver via the portal vein where they are immediately reused. This process of enterohepatic circulation of bile salts is normally very efficient, ensuring there are always adequate bile salts to digest a large meal.

The small intestine is therefore intimately involved in the process of digestion and absorption of food. A basic understanding of these processes will help to ensure that the correct drug and dietary therapy is provided when intestinal disease is present. Any condition which physically damages the small intestine or interferes with the production of enzymes from the pancreas or bile from the liver will prevent the animal from assimilating nutrients from the diet. The extent of the interference will be obvious from the clinical signs exhibited by the animal. For example rotavirus infection may cause diarrhoea and anorexia due to the virus damaging the enterocytes at the tips of the villi. However the condition is usually mild and recovery is rapid. Parvovirus, on the other hand, invades the crypt cells as well as the villus cells and causes severe malabsorption and interference with epithelial renewal. This is reflected in the severity of the clinical signs and their longer duration.

In small intestinal lymphosarcoma and chronic small intestinal disease the animal often has a good appetite accompanied by chronic diarrhoea and marked weight loss. This often confuses the owner, who cannot understand how a good appetite and severe weight loss can occur together. These animals have a marked loss in absorptive ability and are starving in the presence of plenty. Identical clinical signs are observed in dogs with exocrine pancreatic insufficiency but for different reasons. In this latter condition there is a deficiency in digestive enzymes so food cannot be adequately digested and is therefore unable to be absorbed.

To a greater or lesser extent in all the above conditions diet plays an important part in therapy. It is obviously important to determine which condition is present in order to determine if digestion or absorption is affected. Specific drug therapy can then be provided together with a suitable veterinary diet. In all the cases described, feeding large amounts of food while the animal has diarrhoea is unlikely to be successful. The first step is usually to starve the animal for 24 or 48 hours and then provide a low-fat highly-digestible diet in small amounts up to three times daily.

The highly-digestible diet is required to reduce the requirement for enzymes and large surface area for absorption, while maintaining a good level of nutrition. Fat is poorly tolerated in all dogs with diarrhoea and bacterial fermentation results in hydroxy fatty acid production which further stimulates intestinal secretion and diarrhoea. Feeding small meals ensures the endogenous processes of digestion and absorption are not over-whelmed, and reduces the risk of diarrhoea recurring.

A specific form of small intestinal disease and malabsorption has been observed in Irish setters which are sensitive to gluten in their diet (Batt et al., 1984). While these animals are fed cereals the chronic diarrhoea and weight loss persist. When a gluten-free diet is fed the clinical signs slowly subside and the animal gains weight. 'Milk allergy' is a commonly diagnosed cause of chronic diarrhoea but is rarely an allergy, rather an intolerance to milk caused by lactase deficiency. When milk is fed to these dogs diarrhoea occurs, but the symptoms rapidly subside when milk is withdrawn from the diet.

## Large intestine

The large intestine starts at the ileocaecocolic junction and continues as the caecum, ascending, transverse and descending colon, rectum and anus (Fig. 1.13). These divisions have practical significance when viewing radiographs or carrying out endoscopic examinations, as they clearly demarcate the various regions of the large intestine.

The sphincter at the terminal part of the ileum controls the movement of chyme into the colon. The caecum is small and has no known function in the dog and cat. The colon is much shorter in carnivores than in herbivores, indicating the different functions of the colon in these species. The rectum is important for the storage of faeces while the two sphincters at the anus control defaecation.

The colon is composed of mucosa, sub-mucosa, muscle layers and outer

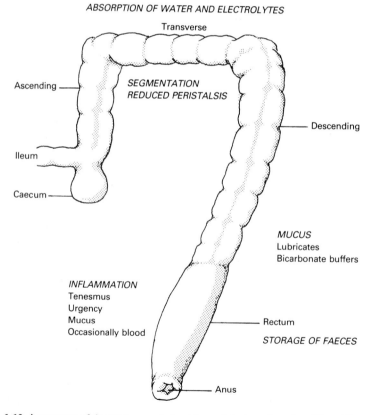

Fig. 1.13 A summary of the anatomy and physiology of the large intestine. (From Simpson & Else, 1991.)

serosa as in the rest of the digestive tract. Unlike the small intestine the mucosa of the colon has a smooth surface with no villi present. There are numerous goblet cells within the mucosa. These cells secrete mucus which lubricates the faeces assisting in their passage to the rectum.

The colon has three functions:

1  The absorption of water and electrolytes.
2  The storage of faeces in the rectum.
3  The fermentation of food residues by a large bacterial population.

To assist in these functions a complex pattern of motility exists which originates from a pacemaker in the mid-colon. Colonic motility is reduced by sympathetic innervation and stimulated by parasympathetic innervation. Following a meal both gastrin and cholecystokinin stimulate colonic motility. Both segmented and peristaltic contractions occur in the colon. The segmented contractions are most prominent in the ascending and transverse colon and are designed to assist in the absorption of water and electrolytes. Retrograde peristalsis against a closed ileal sphincter is also observed in this region, and is also designed to ensure adequate absorption of fluid (Burrows & Merritt, 1983). Powerful peristaltic contractions eventually sweep the remaining colonic contents via the descending colon towards the rectum where the faeces are stored.

Distension of the colon is a powerful stimulant of normal colonic motility and this is best achieved by adding fibre to the diet. Restoration of normal colonic motility by administering fibre can be a satisfactory means of treating both constipation and large intestinal diarrhoea.

No significant digestion or absorption of food occurs in the colon, as this is almost entirely carried out by the small intestine. However the absorption of water and electrolyte from the colon is of great importance in maintaining homeostasis.

The absorption of water by the large intestine is very important in ensuring the passage of formed faeces and preventing dehydration. This assumes even greater importance in cases of small intestinal diarrhoea when the colonic reserve capacity helps to prevent excess fluid loss. Normally, water is passively absorbed from the colon following the active energy-dependent absorption of sodium chloride. This latter process creates very large concentration gradients between the lumen and the mucosal cells which permits the passive movement of water into the cells. This concentration gradient is further enhanced by the bacterial production of volatile fatty acids and ammonia which are absorbed into the mucosal cells. The tight junctions between the cells are very efficient and very little water is able to leak back into the lumen.

If the colon becomes physically damaged or inflamed these mechanisms often fail, and the colon becomes more permeable with movement of water back into the lumen. The active process of salt movement into the mucosal cells may also fail so the concentration gradient is also lost. This further reduces the movement of water into the mucosal cells.

In addition, inflammation may also interfere with colonic motility and lead to a failure in segmentation in the ascending and transverse colon. Often peristalsis is retained. This reduces the amount of mixing of colonic contents and the time spent in the proximal colon, both of which result in less water and salt absorption. Often fluid faecal material is swept towards the rectum before adequate absorption has taken place, resulting in urgency of defaecation and passage of fluid faeces. This has often been misdiagnosed as increased intestinal motility when in fact there is reduced segmentation and normal peristalsis.

Where small intestinal disease is present there may be a failure in bile salt absorption in the ileum as well as inadequate fat digestion and absorption. When these components reach the colon, bacterial fermentation produces deconjugated bile salts and hydroxy fatty acids; both of these products stimulate fluid secretion in the colon adding to the diarrhoea (Binder, 1973).

Bacteria in the colon produce large amounts of ammonia from food residues which are high in nitrogen. This is absorbed and passes into the portal blood and is normally efficiently absorbed by the liver where it is converted to urea and excreted by the kidney. Where congenital or acquired (cirrhosis) liver disease is present, the ammonia remains in the general circulation causing serious central nervous disturbances called hepato-encephalopathy. Treatment of this condition usually involves feeding a low-protein diet of high digestibility together with the provision of drugs to suppress colonic bacterial activity.

Treatment of colitis usually involves the use of sulphasalazine which is taken orally and remains inactive until it reaches the colon. Bacteria in the colon split the drug into a sulphonamide and 5-amino salicyclic acid. It is generally thought that the latter is the active ingredient acting as a non-steroidal anti-inflammatory drug. Dietary management of colitis is subject to some debate. Some workers suggest a highly-digestible low-fat diet which leaves very little residue and so less work for the colon to perform, whereas others suggest a high-fibre diet is important in restoring normal colonic motility. At this time no definitive evidence has been produced to indicate which diet is more effective, although the reasons for suggesting each are understandable. More research is required in this important area.

# References

Argenzio, R.A. (1980) Comparative physiology of the gastrointestinal system. In *Veterinary Gastroenterology*, pp. 172–198. Anderson, N.V. (ed.). Lea & Febiger, Philadelphia.
Batt, R.M., Carter, M.W. & McLean, L. (1984) Morphological and biochemical studies of a

naturally occuring enteropathy in the Irish setter; a comparison with coeliac disease in man. *Research in Veterinary Science*, 37, 339–346.

Binder, H.J. (1973) Faecal fatty acids – mediators of diarrhoea. *Gastroenterology*, 65, 847–850.

Burrows, C.F. & Merritt, A.M. (1983) The influence of alpha cellulose on the myoelectrical activity of the proximal canine colon. *American Journal of Physiology*, 245, G301–G306.

Eastwood, G.L. (1977) Gastrointestinal epithelial renewal. *Gastroenterology*, 72, 962–975.

Evans, H.E. & Christensen, G.C. (1979) The digestive system and abdomen. In *Millers' Anatomy of the Dog*, pp. 411–506. W.B. Saunders, Philadelphia.

Hunt, J.N. & Stubbs, D.F. (1975) The volume and energy content of meals as determinants of gastric emptying. *Journal of Physiology*, 245, 209–225.

McDonald, P., Edwards, R.A. & Greenhaugh, J.F.D. (1988) Digestion. In *Animal Nutrition*, 4th edn, pp. 130–157. Longman Scientific & Technical, Harlow.

Simpson, J.W. & Doxey, D.L. (1983) Quantitative assessment of fat absorption and its diagnostic value in exocrine pancreatic insufficiency. *Research in Veterinary Science*, 35, 249–251.

Simpson, J.W., Doxey, D.L. & Brown, R. (1984) Serum isoamylase values in normal dogs and dogs with exocrine pancreatic insufficiency. *Veterinary Research Communications*, 8, 303–308.

Simpson, J.W. & Else, R.L. (1991) Conditions of the stomach. In *Digestive Disease in the Dog and Cat*, pp. 60–87. Blackwell Scientific Publications, Oxford.

Tennant, B.C. & Hornbuckle, W.E. (1980) Gastrointestinal function. In *Clinical Biochemistry of Domestic Animals*, pp. 283–337. Kaneko, J.J. (ed.). Academic Press, New York.

Tobey, M., Heizer, W., Yek, R., Haang, T. & Hefner, C. (1985) Human intestinal brush border peptidases. *Gastroenterology*, 88, 913–926.

Walsh, J.H., Csendes, A. & Grossman, M.I. (1972) Effects of truncal vagotomy on gastrin release and Heidenheim pouch acid secretion in response to feeding in dogs. *Gastroenterology*, 63, 593–599.

Weber, J. & Kohatsu, M.D. (1970) Pacemaker localiation and electrical conduction patterns in the canine stomach. *Gastroenterology*, 59, 717–726.

# 2 / Nutrients and the Requirements of Dogs and Cats

## Introduction

All living creatures must take in food in order to sustain and generate life. Food may supply materials that can be used by the body to generate energy, materials that can be used in processes such as growth or repair of tissues, and substances which can regulate metabolic activity. The components of the food that perform these functions are known as nutrients, the major classes of which are proteins, fats, carbohydrates, vitamins and minerals.

Each of these broad classes or groups of nutrients is made up of many different substances, and animals often have grossly different requirements for individual nutrients from each of the groups. For example, dogs under normal circumstances can make vitamin C in their bodies, and therefore, do not need it supplied in their diet. Conversely man and the guinea pig lack the mechanism for manufacturing vitamin C, and must find it in their food or suffer the consequences of scurvy. Cats need a supply of preformed taurine in their diets whereas dogs can manufacture sufficient to meet their requirements. The purpose of this chapter is to examine in more detail each of the individual classes of nutrients in relation to the specific needs of dogs and cats.

## Carbohydrates

Each of the members of this group of compounds contains the elements carbon, hydrogen and oxygen. The latter two elements are usually present in the same ratio as in water, i.e. two hydrogen to one oxygen, thus giving rise to the name carbohydrate, or hydrated carbon. Carbohydrates mainly act as an energy source, but may also be converted into body fat and stored, or may serve as starting materials for the metabolism of other compounds. Carbohydrates are conveniently classified into four main groups.

### Monosaccharides

These are represented by a single molecule of what are generically called sugars, which is a little confusing because 'sugar' (sucrose) is actually a disaccharide consisting of one molecule of glucose and one of fructose. The most common monosaccharides are glucose and fructose (found in honey), but there are many others. Monosaccharides can combine with one another to form polymers, and these can be enormous molecules containing many thousands of individual monosaccharide units. This ability to polymerize forms the basis for the classification of carbohydrates.

### Disaccharides

The simplest possible polymer that a monosaccharide can form is one which contains only two molecules, hence disaccharide. The commonest disaccharide to be found in nature is sucrose, but maltose and lactose are also frequently encountered.

### Oligosaccharides

These consist of between 3–10 monosaccharide units, which may be of one type, or of a mixture of different types. They are often difficult to digest, and if found in quantity, particularly as in some plant materials, may be associated with gastro-intestinal disturbances or flatus.

### Polysaccharides

These consist of many thousands of monosaccharide units. They are found widely in plants, and are commonly used as cell wall material (cellulose), or as stores of energy, e.g. starch and glycogen (the carbohydrate reserve of animals). Other common polysaccharides are pectins and hemicelluloses. Complex carbohydrates of plant origin other than starch are referred to as dietary fibre, or non-starch polysaccharides.

Carbohydrate is physiologically essential to the dog and cat, however, it is not essential in the diet of either species provided that the protein level is high enough to supply sufficient gluconeogenic amino acids to allow the maintenance of plasma glucose. Not withstanding this, carbohydrates are a useful source of dietary energy, and provided starch is cooked it is generally readily digested by dogs and cats. Cooking is necessary to break down starch granules. The dog in particular is well able to digest starch, although quantities greater than approximately 65% of the total diet should be avoided.

However, other polysaccharides, such as cellulose, are not utilized and certain disaccharides may also be less well tolerated. The ability to digest lactose, for example, depends on the level of activity of β-galactosidase in the intestine, and whilst present in the adult animals the level of activity of the enzyme is known to be higher in kittens. Lactose intolerance (characterized by diarrhoea) may thus be seen in animals suddenly given amounts of lactose beyond their digestive capabilities. Although individual variations in tolerance must be expected, digestive disorders have been reported in adult dogs with intakes greater than 0.6–1 g lactose/kg body weight/day. This is equivalent to about 10–20 ml of milk/kg body weight daily.

Whilst there have been some suggestions that carbohydrate-free high-fat diets may be advantageous in dogs undergoing very high levels of physical activity, for normal dogs it is acceptable for carbohydrate to provide 40–50% of the total energy in the diet. For cats, a lower level is preferable, and carbohydrate should probably be limited to no more than 30% of dietary energy.

## Lipids

The property most commonly associated with lipids, or fats, is their lack of affinity for water. The majority of lipid in food is in the form of triglycerides, although other types include phospholipids, fat-soluble vitamins and sterols. Triglycerides are compounds of glycerol and three fatty acids, which may be the same or different, and the differences between one fatty acid and another are largely responsible for the differences between triglycerides. The fatty acids have chains of carbon atoms as their backbone, and they can be saturated or unsaturated (presence of one or more double bonds). Saturated and unsaturated fatty acids are found in both animals and plants (Table 2.1).

Dietary fat is important to dogs and cats, as it provides both the most concentrated source of energy, and also texture and flavour to food which are important adjuncts to palatability. Both species normally digest it well. However, establishing a precise requirement for fat is difficult, as the only demonstrable need is to provide essential fatty acids (EFAs) and to act

**Table 2.1** Some examples of fatty acids

| Fatty acid | Saturated | Unsaturated | Source |
|---|---|---|---|
| Butyric acid | Fully | – | Butter |
| Palmitic acid | Fully | – | Vegetable oils, animal fats |
| Stearic acid | Fully | – | Animal fats, vegetable oils |
| Oleic acid | – | One double bond | Vegetable oils, animal fats |
| Linoleic acid | – | Two double bonds | Vegetable oils |
| Linolenic acid | – | Three double bonds | Vegetable oils |
| Arachidonic acid | – | Four double bonds | Small quantities in selected animal fats |

Vegetable oils are often artificially hydrogenated to convert them into a saturated fat, for example, margarine.

as a carrier for fat-soluble vitamins. Recognized EFAs include linoleic, α-linolenic, and arachidonic acids. The first two of these are parent compounds for the more complex derived EFAs that can be synthesized in the body. EFAs are essential to the health of the animal and deficiency (see p. 47) is associated with a wide range of clinical problems. They form part of the structure of cell membranes and act as precursors for the biosynthesis of a variety of potent short lived compounds, the eicosanoids, which have a wide variety of functions, including a major role in the induction and modulation of inflammation.

In the dog a requirement has been established for linoleic acid, and it is assumed that a requirement also exists for α-linolenic acid, although this has yet to be determined. In common with most mammals it does not require a dietary source of arachidonic acid. An important difference exists in this respect between the cat and the dog. It has been reported that the cat has limited activity of certain desaturase enzymes involved in EFA metabolism, and a dietary requirement for a derived EFA, arachidonic acid, has been established for this species. In practical terms this means a requirement for animal fat in the diet, and thus this is one of the factors contributing to the nature of the cat as an obligate carnivore.

## Protein

Proteins are very complex molecules and are universal and indispensable constituents of every living organism. A complex animal such as a dog or a cat possesses a very large number of individual proteins, in fact probably around 60 000 of them. All of these proteins are polymers composed of only about 20 different α-amino acids. Proteins are formed by the amino group of one amino acid joining with the acid group of another; such a linkage is known as a peptide bond. Through this mechanism hundreds (or perhaps thousands) of amino acids can be joined in a variety of sequences to give rise to the range of proteins that occur in nature.

In addition to the nitrogen in their amino group some amino acids also contain sulphur, consequently chemical analysis of a protein will yield carbon, hydrogen, oxygen, nitrogen and sulphur as the main constituents. Proteins can also become bonded to other molecules, and this is a useful basis for a relatively simple classification.

### Simple proteins

On hydrolysis these give rise to their constituent amino acids only. Examples include:

1 *Albumins* are globular proteins found in egg white, blood plasma and milk.

**2** *Collagens* are fibrous proteins present in connective tissue, and converted to gelatin on prolonged boiling.

**3** *Elastins* are fibrous elastic proteins found in artery walls and skin.

*Conjugated proteins*

On hydrolysis these yield other distinctive substances in addition to amino acids. When coupled with the protein these are called the prosthetic groups. Examples include:

**1** *Glycoproteins* contain carbohydrate, e.g. mucus.

**2** *Lipoproteins* contain lipid, involved with fat transport in blood and in cell wall formation.

**3** *Phosphoproteins* contain a phosphate group, the most well known being casein in milk.

**4** *Chromoproteins* contain a pigment group, for example haem in haemoglobin.

**5** *Nucleoproteins* combine proteins and nucleic acids, which together are involved in cell division and the transfer of heritable characteristics in the cell nucleus as genes.

Protein is required by dogs and cats to provide a source of amino acids to build, repair and replace their body proteins. Amino acids are divided into two groups, non-essential and essential. The term non-essential is perhaps unfortunate, as the amino acids concerned are just as important in the proteins as the essential group; the distinction between the two is that the latter must be available from the diet, whereas the former can be synthesized by the body from other precursors at a rate sufficient to meet physiological needs.

The protein and essential amino acid requirements of the dog and cat have been studied in considerable detail (Tables 2.2 and 2.3), and another important nutritional difference emerges in that it has been established that the cat has a higher requirement for protein than the dog. This has been shown not to be due to a higher requirement for essential amino acids, but rather because some of the nitrogen catabolic enzymes of the cat are permanently set to handle a high level of dietary protein, and their activity is not modified even when the cat is receiving a low protein diet.

Many of the experiments into the protein and amino acid requirements of dogs and cats have been conducted using semi-purified diets. Care should be taken when extrapolating data from these studies to practical feeding situations, as the amino acid profiles and digestibility of naturally occurring protein sources need to be taken into account. In general, animal protein sources will have a better amino acid profile and digestibility than plant sources. The recommendations given in Table 2.2 take account of the typical digestibilities and amino acid profiles of the types of foods likely to be fed to dogs and cats.

Table 2.2 Recommended minimum nutrient levels in dog and cat diets. (After Burger, 1988.)

| Nutrient | Dogs | Cats |
|---|---|---|
| Protein (g)* | 22 | 28 |
| Fat (g)† | 5.5 | 9.0 |
| Linoleic and arachidonic acids (g)† | 1.1 | 1.0 |
| Arachidonic acid alone (g)† | – | 0.02 |
| Calcium (g) | 1.1 | 1.0 |
| Phosphorus (g) | 0.9 | 0.8 |
| Ca:P ratio | 0.8–1.5:1 | 0.8–1.5:1 |
| Sodium (g) | 0.08 | 0.2 |
| Potassium (g) | 0.5 | 0.5 |
| Magnesium (g) | 0.04 | 0.05 |
| Iron (mg)‡ | 8.0 | 10 |
| Copper (mg)‡ | 0.7 | 0.5 |
| Manganese (mg)‡ | 0.5 | 1.0 |
| Zinc (mg)‡ | 5.0 | 4.0 |
| Iodine (mg) | 0.15 | 0.1 |
| Selenium (µg) | 10 | 10 |
| Vitamin A (IU) | 500 | 550 |
| Vitamin D (IU) | 50 | 100 |
| Vitamin E (mg)† | 5.0 | 8.0 |
| Vitamin K (µg)§ | 8.0 | 10 |
| Thiamin (mg) | 0.1 | 0.5 |
| Riboflavin (mg) | 0.25 | 0.5 |
| Pantothenic acid (mg) | 1.1 | 1.0 |
| Niacin (mg) | 1.2 | 4.5 |
| Pyridoxine (mg) | 0.12 | 0.4 |
| Folic acid (µg)§ | 22 | 100 |
| Vitamin $B_{12}$ (µg) | 2.7 | 2.0 |
| Choline (mg) | 125 | 200 |
| Biotin (mg)§ | 0.05 | 0.007 |
| Taurine (mg)¶ | – | 100 or 250 |

Values expressed per 400 kcal (1.7 MJ) metabolizable energy (ME), which approximates to 100 g dry matter (DM) in typical commercial pet foods.
* Protein levels assume a balanced amino acid profile and satisfactory digestibility.
† Fat content stated only as a guide. Key nutrients are the EFA linoleic and arachidonic acids. With high levels of EFA, vitamin E will need to be increased.
‡ Figures assume high availability. Particularly important to ensure that this is the case with these nutrients.
§ A dietary requirement for these nutrients has not been demonstrated when natural ingredients were fed. This is because intestinal bacterial synthesis can meet the needs of the animal. Supplementation may be necessary if anti-bacterial or anti-vitamin compounds are being administered or present in the diet.
¶ 100 mg/400 kcal for dry foods, 250 mg/400 kcal for canned foods.

## Taurine

Before completing this section on proteins special mention should be made of taurine, because of its particular nutritional significance to the cat. Taurine is not an α-amino acid, and therefore does not form part of the polypeptide chains that make up proteins. It belongs to a separate group of amino acids, called amino-sulphonic acids.

**Table 2.3** Essential amino acid requirements of the growing dog and cat

| Amino acid | Dog* | Cat* |
|---|---|---|
| Arginine | 1.37 | 2.0 |
| Histidine | 0.49 | 0.6 |
| Isoleucine | 0.98 | 1.0 |
| Leucine | 1.59 | 2.4 |
| Lysine | 1.40 | 1.6 |
| Methionine + cystine | 1.06 | 1.5 |
| Phenylalanine + tyrosine | 1.95 | 1.7 |
| Threonine | 1.27 | 1.4 |
| Tryptophan | 0.41 | 0.3 |
| Valine | 1.05 | 1.2 |
| Total | 11.57 | 13.7 |

* Amount required: g/1000 kcal of ME (1 kcal = 4.184 kJ).
Data reprinted with permission from *Nutrient Requirements of Dogs*, © 1985, and *Nutrient Requirements of Cats*, © 1986 by the National Academy of Sciences. Published by National Academy Press, Washington, DC.

**Table 2.4** Taurine content of some foods

| Item | Taurine content: mg/100 g wet weight |
|---|---|
| Beef (round)* | 15–47 |
| Beef (liver)* | 14–27 |
| Lamb (leg)* | 45–51 |
| Lamb (kidney)* | 13–44 |
| Lamb (muscle)† | 62–106 |
| Pork (loin)* | 39–69 |
| Chicken (leg)* | 30–38 |
| Chicken (muscle)† | 15–16 |
| Rabbit (muscle)† | 24–32 |
| Cod (frozen)* | 23–40 |
| Oysters (fresh)* | 39–124 |
| Clams (fresh)* | 145–370 |

* From Roe & Weston (1965), reprinted by permission from *Nature*, **205**, 287–288, © 1965 Macmillan Magazines Ltd.
† From Wills (1991), reprinted by permission from *In Practice*, **13**, 87–93, © 1991 British Veterinary Association.

It has been shown comparatively recently that taurine is an essential nutrient for the cat, and that dietary deficiency is linked with several important conditions (see p. 51). The cat's particular dietary requirement for taurine arises from its limited ability to synthesize taurine from sulphur-containing animo acids, and from its handling of taurine in bile acid conjugation. The latter is important as the cat appears not to produce bile salts conjugated with glycine even in times of taurine deficiency, and thus does not 'spare' taurine via this route. This combination of factors makes the cat particularly susceptible to a dietary deficiency of taurine.

Taurine is present in a range of meats and seafoods (Table 2.4), but is essentially absent from plant materials, and thus the cat's requirement for this nutrient is another example of factors making it an obligate carnivore.

A further twist to the taurine story occurred in 1987 when it was established that levels of taurine in some foods which were previously considered adequate, could actually be associated with taurine deficiency in the cat. As a result of this, different recommendations are now made for the taurine content of different types of food (Table 2.2). The underlying mechanism for the higher requirement associated with the feeding of canned foods has yet to be established, although it is the subject of current research. It is likely that manufacturers of commercial foods will now have adjusted taurine levels in their recipes to values similar to those given.

## Minerals

All animals require a variety of inorganic materials in their diets. Some minerals are required in relatively large quantities because they form a major part of the body's structural elements, for example, calcium in bone. Others, which are used in the chemical processes of metabolism, may only be required in minute traces.

The minerals for which requirements have (to date) been established in the dog or cat are relatively few and include calcium, phosphorus, magnesium, sodium, potassium, chlorine, iron, zinc, copper, iodine, manganese and selenium. Many more, for example silicon, arsenic, nickel and molybdenum are usually found on analysis, but although functions have been established for these in some mammals, specific requirements have not been established for the dog and cat. Actually, it is not surprising that many other elements are found, since several of them are very widely distributed in nature, and are therefore likely to be ingested in the normal course of eating. Provided they remain at trace levels they do no demonstrable harm. However, it should be remembered that even those minerals which are known to be essential are often toxic in excess, and consequently their intake through the diet or through supplementation must be carefully regulated. For a diet which is known to be nutritionally complete in its mineral content, further supplementation is at best wasteful, and at worst injurious to the health of the animal.

### Calcium and phosphorus

Although these two elements do have separate functions within the body, they are so closely interrelated that they are usually considered together. The vast majority of body calcium and phosphorus (around 99% and 85% respectively) is found in bones and teeth. These minerals have a range of functions apart from their role in structure. Calcium is involved in blood clotting, nerve and muscle function. Phosphorus has a wide variety of other functions, actually more than any other mineral in the body. It is involved in many enzyme systems and is, for example, essential for the utilization of energy from food.

Dietary recommendations have been established for calcium and phosphorus for dogs and cats, but in addition the ratio between the two is of particular importance, and imbalances in this ratio as well as deficiencies of calcium or phosphorus can be associated with health problems (see p. 43). The optimal calcium to phosphorus ratio for growing dogs and cats is considered to lie between 0.8 : 1 and 1.5 : 1.

Many dog owners, particularly those with puppies of the large and giant breeds, like to supplement the diets of their pets with either calcium, or a combination of calcium and phosphorus. Whilst this is appropriate if the diet is deficient (such as a diet based on fresh meat), it is not only unnecessary, but potentially dangerous if the diet already contains adequate levels of these minerals. A commonly used calcium and phosphorus supplement is bone meal. Most bone meal preparations contain about 30% calcium and 15% phosphorus. If diets are fed which are based mainly on lean meats this may be used as a supplement, and about 7 g should be added per 450 g of meat to balance the calcium and phosphorus levels. Care should be taken not to oversupplement, as skeletal problems have been reported in dogs on intakes as low as three times those recommended.

### Potassium, sodium and chloride

These three minerals are largely found in body fluids and soft tissues. Sodium and chloride are the major electrolytes of the extracellular fluid, whereas 98% of body potassium is intracellular. Potassium, sodium and chloride are involved in maintaining osmotic pressure, acid–base equilibria, and in controlling water balance. Potassium and sodium are also important in neural and muscular function. Dietary recommendations have been established for the dog and cat, but as these minerals are widely distributed in nature, a simple deficiency of any of them is likely to be rare.

Hypokalaemic polymyopathy has, however, been observed in cats under specific circumstances. Increased dietary potassium to above the recommendations given in Table 2.2 is advisable in diets designed for urinary acidification, or for cats with renal failure.

### Magnesium

Magnesium is mainly present in bone and muscle, although it also occurs in other tissues. In addition to its role as a constituent of bones and teeth, magnesium is also essential for a wide range of cellular reactions, including those concerned with energy metabolism. Magnesium is widespread in foods, especially those of vegetable origin, and thus a dietary deficiency is unlikely to occur. High dietary intakes of magnesium have been linked with an increased risk of certain types of lower urinary tract disease in cats, due to an increase in the risk of struvite (magnesium ammonium phosphate) formation. This is discussed in more detail in Chapter 4.

### Trace elements

Brief notes on the function of some trace elements are given in Table 2.5. A detailed discussion of the functions of each of these is beyond the scope of

**Table 2.5** Summary of functions of some trace elements. (After Burger, 1988.)

| Element | Function |
|---------|----------|
| Cobalt | Component of vitamin $B_{12}$; none may be required by the dog or cat if intake of $B_{12}$ is adequate |
| Copper | Component of many enzyme systems; linked with iron metabolism, and therefore haemoglobin synthesis; involved in maintenance of structural integrity of bones and blood vessels; necessary for melanin production |
| Iodine | Constituent of thyroid hormones |
| Iron | Component of haemoglobin and myoglobin and a number of enzymes including those essential for oxygen utilization at the cellular level |
| Manganese | Component of various enzyme systems; necessary for chondroitin sulphate and cholesterol biosynthesis; involved in some aspects of carbohydrate and fat metabolism |
| Selenium | Component of glutathione peroxidase; acts with vitamin E to protect cell membranes from oxidative damage |
| Zinc | Component of many enzymes (60 or more) including RNA polymerase (hence role in protein biosynthesis), alkaline phosphatase, carbonic anhydrase, and some digestive enzymes |
| Chromium | Carbohydrate metabolism, closely linked with insulin function |
| Fluoride | Teeth and bone development, possibly some involvement in reproduction |
| Nickel | Membrane function, possibly involved in metabolism of the nucleic acid RNA |
| Molybdenum | Constituent of several enzymes, one of which is involved in uric acid metabolism |
| Silicon | Skeletal development, growth and maintenance of connective tissue |
| Vanadium | Growth, reproduction, fat metabolism |
| Arsenic | Growth, also some effect on blood formation, possibly haemoglobin production |

this chapter, and is covered by other standard texts (see Further reading). Dietary recommendations have been established for some trace minerals in the dog and cat (see Table 2.2), but not for others which are known to be necessary for health in other mammals. It is likely that this latter group are required only in very small amounts, and that deficiency with normal diets is highly unlikely. However, as noted earlier the potential for toxicity exists with these trace elements as it does for other minerals if the intake is excessive, although the toxicity of individual minerals varies.

## Vitamins

The vitamins are a diverse group of nutrients which are not united by any common chemical or physical grouping. They are, however, united in their disparity, in that vitamins are a group of individual organic compounds of which small quantities are essential to life. They are associated with the metabolism of other nutrients and with maintaining the body's normal physiological functioning. They are found in differing quantities in foods, but no one food, unless specially prepared from a mixture of ingredients, has all of them in sufficient quantity to satisfy the body's needs. Rather like the trace elements, vitamins are only required in small quantities, and what is an essential vitamin for one species may not be so for another, the case of vitamin C being essential for man, but not for the dog, having already been cited.

Vitamins have come into prominence mainly because of the problems associated with deficiencies. Thus they were often discovered as absences, such as in the diseases of beriberi, pellagra, pernicious anaemia and rickets. Following the identification of the dietary relationship to disease, later scientists have been able to isolate, identify and even to manufacture vitamins.

Vitamins are often classified into two major categories on the basis of whether they are water- or fat-soluble. Thus the fat-soluble vitamins A, D, E and K are found in foods associated with lipids, and are absorbed along with dietary fat. They can be stored in the body and consequently a dog or cat is not absolutely dependent on a daily supply. In general, water-soluble vitamins are not stored in significant quantities, excesses being excreted in urine. Thus they are usually required in daily quantities in the diet.

### Fat-soluble vitamins

*Vitamin A*

Vitamin A is a term which describes several compounds which biologically have the activity of the parent compound retinol. This form of the vitamin and its derivatives are found only in animal tissues, whereas plants contain precursors in the form of the carotenoids, the yellow/orange pigments found in carrots and many other vegetables. The most widely abundant precursor of vitamin A is β-carotene, and most animals can convert this into the vitamin itself. The best known function for vitamin A is the role it plays in vision. The vitamin combines with the protein opsin to create rhodopsin. This in turn is split on exposure to light giving rise to a series of reactions leading to the generation of nerve impulses. One manifestation of vitamin A deficiency is thus slow dark adaptation, progressing to night blindness. Vitamin A is also involved in many other physiological functions. It is concerned with the normal development of bone, one sign of deficiency being retardation of bone growth. It is essential for the normal maintenance of epithelial tissue, and may also be involved in spermatogenesis and foetal development.

Fish liver oils are the most concentrated source of vitamin A, but animal liver, egg yolk and kidney are also good sources. Within plants, variable amounts of β-carotene are found in carrots and dark green or yellow vegetables. The potency of fish liver oils as vitamin A (and D) supplements means that they should only be used with great care. Typically, cod liver oil contains 18 mg of retinol, 0.21 mg of vitamin D and 20 mg of vitamin E per 100 g. One teaspoonful (about 5 g) would provide all the daily vitamin A and D requirements for an adult 50 kg dog.

Another important nutritional difference exists between the cat and the dog with regard to dietary sources of vitamin A. The cat lacks the ⟨ necessary to cleave β-carotene, and is thus dependent on a dietary s⟨ preformed vitamin A. Preformed vitamin A, as noted above, is restr⟨ animal tissues, and thus this is another factor contributing to the ⟨ carnivore status of the cat.

*Vitamin D*

Again the term vitamin D covers a number of related compounds which have activity associated with vitamin D, the two most important of which are vitamin $D_2$ (ergocalciferol) and $D_3$ (cholecalciferol). Biochemical conversion of vitamin D occurs in the liver and kidney to produce physiologically active (dihydroxylated) forms of the vitamin. Vitamin D is involved in a number of aspects of calcium and phosphorus metabolism, and its overall effect is to increase net retention of these minerals and bring about mineralization of bone. This is accomplished through indirect effects in the gastro-intestinal tract, increasing absorption of calcium and phosphorus; on the kidney decreasing the excretion of calcium and phosphorus; and on bone where it has two effects, increased mineralization as well as increased bone reabsorption.

There is some debate about the vitamin D requirements of dogs and cats. Most mammals can form vitamin $D_3$ in the skin after exposure to ultraviolet (UV) light, thereby sparing a dietary requirement. In addition, it is likely in dogs and cats that the requirement may also be influenced by the dietary calcium and phosphorus content and ratio. Although rickets has been produced experimentally in growing kittens, more recently it has been reported that the vitamin D requirement appears to be extremely low, provided that a diet with a correct calcium:phosphorus ratio and adequate levels of these minerals is fed, even if the cats are shielded from UV light. The situation with dogs appears more complex, and although again it is likely that the vitamin D requirement may be low when diets with correct mineral composition are fed, rickets has been reported in dogs fed vitamin D deficient (but otherwise adequate) diets even when exposed to UV light. This suggests that unlike many other mammals, the dog does not synthesize adequate vitamin D in its skin and, therefore, requires a dietary source. Recommendations for the vitamin D content of diets are given in Table 2.2.

## Vitamin E

Vitamin E includes a number of compounds, of which the most biologically active and widely distributed is α-tocopherol. Vitamin E functions as an important anti-oxidant within cells, protecting lipids, particularly the polyunsaturated fatty acids (PUFA) in cell membranes, against oxidative damage caused by free radicals and active forms of oxygen that may be generated during metabolic processes.

The dietary requirement for vitamin E is influenced by the intake of selenium (because of its role in glutathione peroxidase), with one nutrient partially able to spare a deficiency of the other. It is also influenced by the PUFA content of the diet, and increasing this leads to an increase in vitamin E requirement. It has been recommended that a dietary ratio of α-tocopherol:PUFA (mg/g) of 0.6:1 is maintained as a minimum to protect against PUFA peroxidation. Rancid fats are particularly destructive of vitamin E, so these should be avoided in diets.

## Vitamin K

There are several quinone type compounds that have vitamin K activity. Vitamin K is required for normal blood clotting, as it is needed for the production of normal prothrombin and for the synthesis of clotting factors VII, IX and X. Deficiency is, therefore, characterized by increased clotting time.

A simple dietary deficiency of vitamin K is unlikely to occur in dogs and cats under normal circumstances, as they can obtain much (if not all) of their requirement for the vitamin from intestinal bacterial synthesis. Thus it is only if this is suppressed, for example with anti-bacterial therapy, or if the absorption or function of vitamin K is interfered with, that a dietary supply becomes necessary. Recommended allowances for vitamin K are given in Table 2.2.

## Water-soluble vitamins

The water-soluble vitamins that are important in nutrition of the dog and cat are members of the B complex. They are used by the animal to form coenzymes which function in a variety of important reactions including the oxidation of amino acids, fatty acids and carbohydrates and in certain biosynthetic reactions. A coenzyme is a molecule that binds to a protein (the apoenzyme) to produce an active enzyme (holoenzyme). They represent one type of cofactor, the other being a metal ion, examples of which have already been discussed in this chapter. Coenzymes usually function as carriers of molecules or parts of molecules that are transferred in enzymatic reactions.

### Thiamin (B₁)

Thiamin is converted in the liver to thiamin pyrophosphate which then acts as a key coenzyme in carbohydrate metabolism. Thus the thiamin requirement of an animal is influenced by the carbohydrate content of its diet, and a high-fat, low-carbohydrate diet will result in a lower requirement. Thiamin deficiency will result in impairment of carbohydrate metabolism and accumulation of pyruvic and lactic acids within the body, leading to clinical signs (see p. 48).

Thiamin is widely distributed in foods, good sources being brewer's yeast, whole cereal grains, organ meats and egg yolk. However, the vitamin is heat labile and is progressively destroyed by cooking. This problem is normally overcome in commercial foods by supplementing with a sufficiently large quantity preprocessing to take account of any losses, thus ensuring that the finished product meets or exceeds the requirement of the animal.

In common with other water-soluble vitamins thiamin has a very low oral toxicity.

### Riboflavin (B₂)

Riboflavin is a constituent of a number of enzyme systems. Flavin mononucleotide and flavin-adenine-dinucleotide (the coenzyme forms of this vitamin) are necessary for a number of oxidative enzyme systems and thus are needed in every living cell. Riboflavin is more stable to heat than thiamin, but is sensitive to light.

Some of the requirement for this vitamin may be met by intestinal microbial synthesis, however, the contribution that this makes to the requirement of dogs and cats is not known, and a dietary supply is considered essential. Significant sources of this vitamin are to be found in liver, kidney and milk.

## Niacin

The term niacin includes nicotinic acid and nicotinamide. Both compounds are stable to heat and light and hence within foods. The vitamin is widely distributed in foods, with the main sources meats, liver and fish. However, niacin present in maize and some other cereals is largely present in a bound form which is unavailable. Niacin is incorporated into two important coenzymes (nicotinamide-adenine-dinucleotide and its phosphate), which are involved in key steps in the metabolism of protein, fat and carbohydrate.

In the dog the requirement for niacin is influenced by the level of tryptophan in the diet, as this can be converted to niacin, a process not available to the cat. This nutritional difference is not the result of a specific enzyme lack, indeed the cat does possess all the necessary enzymes, but is due to a high level of activity of the enzyme picolinic carboxylase, which effectively diverts tryptophan conversion via an alternative pathway away from niacin. It has been suggested that the high level of activity of picolinic carboxylase may actually protect the cat against the toxic effects of the ingestion of high levels of tryptophan which would accompany its carnivorous diet. Dietary recommendations for niacin are given in Table 2.2.

## Pyridoxine (B₆)

There are three related components with vitamin $B_6$ activity, pyridoxine, pyridoxal and pyridoxamine. All three are convertible in the animal to pyridoxal phosphate which is the active coenzyme. This coenzyme is involved in a wide range of enzyme systems particularly associated with amino acid metabolism. For example, one of the steps in the conversion of tryptophan to niacin is pyridoxal dependent, as is the production of neuro-active amines such as serotonin and γ-aminobutyric acid, and it is also involved in the biosynthesis of taurine. Pyridoxine is required by dogs and cats, and a range of deficiency signs have been reported, including irreversible kidney damage in cats associated with deposition of calcium oxalate crystals. The vitamin is widely distributed in foods; yeast, muscle meats, cereal grains and vegetables are good sources.

*Biotin*

Biotin is a sulphur-containing vitamin, which functions as a coenzyme in carboxylases which catalyse the transfer of carboxyl groups. Biotin is essential for a key step in gluconeogenesis, and in the production of energy through the tricarboxylic acid cycle; and for the production of malonyl-CoA, necessary for the synthesis of long chain fatty acids. The vitamin may also play a role in the metabolism of certain amino acids.

Although biotin is required by dogs and cats, the likelihood of a natural deficiency occurring is small, because most (perhaps all), of the requirement may be met by bacterial synthesis. However, suppression of this by antibacterial drugs may increase the dependence upon dietary supplies. In addition, egg white is known to contain a protein called avidin, which forms a stable complex with biotin, preventing the absorption of both biotin supplied in the diet and that synthesized in the intestine. Uncombined avidin is relatively heat labile, and thus eggs should be fed cooked if they constitute a significant part of the diet. However the risks associated with raw egg white should not be overstated; although estimates are not available for the dog, about 20 egg whites per day have been estimated as the number needed to produce biotin deficiency in man.

*Pantothenic acid*

Pantothenic acid is a component of coenzyme A, and is thus involved in the metabolism of carbohydrates, fats and some amino acids. The vitamin is widely distributed in foodstuffs, and a naturally occurring deficiency is most unlikely in dogs and cats, although it has been produced with experimental diets.

*Folic acid (pteroylglutamic acid)*

Folic acid requires enzymatic changes to form the parent compounds (tetrahydrofolyl polyglutamates) from which the folate coenzymes active in the body are derived. These function in various reactions involving the transfer of single carbon atoms. Included are biosynthetic reactions necessary for nucleic acid synthesis and hence cell replication. One sign characteristic of folate deficiency is anaemia, which arises as a consequence of inadequate nucleoprotein formation for blood-cell maturation.

Folic acid is synthesized by bacteria in the intestine and it is likely that this largely meets the daily requirement of the animal under normal circumstances, although deficiency has been produced experimentally by feeding semi-purified diets. Naturally occurring deficiencies would be uncommon.

*Choline*

Choline is a component of the group of phospholipids called lecithins, and is thus an essential component of cell membranes. In addition, it is necessary for the formation of the neurotransmitter acetylcholine; it acts as a lipotropic substance, preventing abnormal accumulation of fat in the liver; and it acts as a source of methyl groups in various metabolic reactions.

The requirement for choline is influenced by the dietary concentration of other methyl donors, particularly methionine, and as with vitamin E and selenium, an increased supply of one will reduce the requirement for the other. This factor, together with the widespread distribution of choline in animal and plant materials means that deficiency is unlikely to occur in cats or dogs.

*Vitamin B$_{12}$*

Vitamin B$_{12}$ has a very complex chemical structure and is the only vitamin that contains a trace element, cobalt. When isolated from natural sources, vitamin B$_{12}$ is usually in the form of cyanocobalamin. When transformed to a metabolically active coenzyme, the cyano group is replaced by another chemical group which is attached to the cobalt.

The function of vitamin B$_{12}$ is closely linked to that of folic acid, and it too is involved in the transmethylation process which is necessary for DNA synthesis, and deficiency is again associated with nutritional anaemia. Vitamin B$_{12}$ is also necessary for the normal functioning of the nervous system, deficiency having been associated with demyelination, and it is also involved in fat and carbohydrate metabolism.

Vitamin B$_{12}$ is absent from plants, as in nature it is only made by microorganisms. Good sources include liver, kidney and heart, although some seafoods can also supply useful amounts. For effective intestinal vitamin B$_{12}$ absorption, a carrier protein called intrinsic factor is needed. This is secreted into the stomach. Without the presence of intrinsic factor, vitamin B$_{12}$ deficiency will occur.

Precise requirements for vitamin B$_{12}$ have not been established for the dog and cat. The recommendations given in Table 2.2 are based on information from other mammals and some data from these species.

*Ascorbic acid (vitamin C)*

Dogs and cats are able to synthesize ascorbic acid and thus do not have a dietary requirement for this vitamin. Nevertheless, ascorbic acid deficiency has been implicated in some skeletal diseases in the dog, notably hypertrophic oesteodystrophy, and decreased plasma ascorbic acid levels have been found in this condition. However, these may be a consequence, and not a cause of disease, and other research has failed to demonstrate benefits of ascorbic acid supplementation. Indeed, one group suggested that the net result of supplementation could only be an aggravation of disease.

One area where vitamin C supplementation may be of value is in dogs subjected to severe physical stress. Studies in racing sledge dogs have suggested that addition of about 1 mg ascorbic acid/kcal (4.184 kJ) of metabolizable energy in the diet appears to help the dogs to cope with stress.

In general, there seems no reason to advocate the addition of ascorbic acid to the diets of normal, healthy, dogs and cats, unless they are under the special conditions described above.

## Dietary recommendations for individual nutrients

The amount of specific nutrients that a dog or cat requires from its diet will be affected by a number of factors including individual variation, physical activity, weight, sex and life stage. The National Research Council of the National Academy of Sciences of the USA publishes minimum nutrient requirements for growth in dogs and cats, but these data require careful interpretation to be used for the practical formulation of diets. This is partly because they are minima, and due allowance should be made for the factors considered above, but also because the availability of nutrients from different foods must be taken into account when actually formulating diets. All of these factors must be considered when making nutrient recommendations to cover a population of animals fed on diets made from normal (as against semi-purified) ingredients. Table 2.2 provides a list of recommended nutrient concentrations for diets designed to be complete and balanced for the growing and breeding animal as well as for adult maintenance. These figures do incorporate assumptions about nutrient availability and amino acid profiles of likely protein sources and type of ingredients. Whilst they cannot provide a guarantee of nutritional quality, they do provide a good guideline for producing a correctly balanced diet.

## Further reading

Bondi, A.A. (1987) *Animal Nutrition.* Wiley & Sons, Chichester.

Brown, M.L., Filer Jr, L.J., Guthrie, H.A., Levander, O.A., McCormick, D.B., Olson, R.E. & Steele, R.D. (eds) (1990) *Present Knowledge in Nutrition*, 6th edn. International Life Sciences Institute Nutrition Foundation, Washington, DC.

Burger, I.H. (1988) A basic guide to nutrient requirements. In *Dog and Cat Nutrition*, 2nd edn, pp. 9–34, Edney, A.T.B. (ed.). Pergamon Press, Oxford.

Donoghue, S., Kronfeld, D.S. & Banta, C.A. (1987) A possible vitamin C requirement in racing sledge dogs trained on a high fat diet. In *Nutrition, Malnutrition and Dietetics in the Dog and Cat*, pp. 57–59, Edney, A.T.B. (ed.). British Veterinary Association, London/

Waltham Centre for Pet Nutrition, Melton Mowbray.

Dow, S.W., Fettman, M.J., Curtis, C.R. & LeCouteur, R.A. (1989) Hypokalaemia in cats: 186 cases (1984–1987). *Journal of the American Veterinary Medical Association*, **194**, 1604–1608.

Georgievskii, V.I., Annenkov, B.N. & Samokhin, V.I. (1982) *Mineral Nutrition of Animals*. Butterworths, London.

Hazewinkel, H.A.W. (1989) Calcium metabolism and skeletal development in dogs. In *Nutrition of the Dog and Cat*, pp. 293–302, Burger, I.H. & Rivers, J.P.W. (eds). Cambridge University Press, Cambridge.

Hazewinkel, H.A.W., How, K.L., Bosch, R., Goedegebuure, S.A. & Voorhout, G. (1987) Inadequate photosynthesis of vitamin D in dogs. In *Nutrition, Malnutrition and Dietetics in the Dog and Cat*, pp. 66–68, Edney, A.T.B. (ed.). British Veterinary Association, London/Waltham Centre for Pet Nutrition, Melton Mowbray.

Ikeda, M., Tsuji, H., Nakamura, S., Ichiyama, A., Nishizuka, Y. & Hayaishi, O. (1965) Studies on the biosynthesis of nicotinamide adenine dinucleotide II. A role of picolinic carboxylase in the biosynthesis of nicotinamide adenine dinucleotide from tryptophan in mammals. *Journal of Biological Chemistry*, **240**, 1395–1401.

Kendall, P. (1980) Too much supplementation may be harmful. *Pedigree Digest*, **7**, 4.

Kronfeld, D.S., Hammel, E.P., Ramberg Jr, C.F. & Dunlop Jr, H.L. (1977) Haematological and metabolic responses to training in racing sled dogs fed diets containing medium, low or zero carbohydrate. *Americal Journal of Clinical Nutrition*, **30**, 419–430.

Kronfeld, D.S. (1982) Feeding dogs for hard work and stress. In *Dog and Cat Nutrition*, pp. 61–73, Edney, A.T.B (ed.). Pergamon Press, Oxford.

McCay, C.M. (1949) *Nutrition of the Dog*. Comstock Publishing Company, Ithaca, NY.

Maynard, L.A. & Loosli, J.K. (1962) *Animal Nutrition*, 5th edn. McGraw-Hill, New York.

Mercer, J.R. & Silva, S.V.P.S. (1989) Tryptophan metabolism in the cat. In *Nutrition of the Dog and Cat*, pp. 207–227, Burger, I.H. & Rivers, J.P.W. (eds). Cambridge University Press, Cambridge.

Meyer, H. (1979) The pathogenesis of nutrition-induced diarrhoea in dogs. In *Diarrhoea in the Dog*, pp. 13–17, Edney, A.T.B. (ed.). Pedigree Petfoods, Melton Mowbray.

Mund, H.-C. & Meyer, H. (1989) Pathogenesis of lactose-induced diarrhoea and its prevention by enzymatic splitting of lactose. In *Nutrition of the Dog and Cat*, pp. 267–274, Burger, I.H. & Rivers, J.P.W. (eds). Cambridge University Press, Cambridge.

National Research Council (1985) *Nutrient Requirements of Dogs*. National Academy Press, Washington, DC.

National Research Council (1986) *Nutrient Requirements of Cats*. National Academy Press, Washington, DC.

Rivers, J.P.W., Frankel, T.L., Juttla, S. & Hay A.W.M. (1979) Vitamin D in the nutrition of the cat. *Proceedings of the Nutrition Society*, **38**, 36A.

Rivers, J.P.W., Sinclair, A.J. & Crawford, M.A. (1975) Inability of the cat to desaturate essential fatty acids. *Nature*, **258**, 171–173.

Roe, D.A. & Weston, M.O. (1965) Potential significance of free taurine in the diet. *Nature*, **205**, 287–288.

Teare, J.A., Hedhammar, A. & Krook, L. (1980) Influence of growth intensity on the skeletal development of dogs: effects of ascorbic acid supplementation. In *Nutrition of the Dog and Cat*, pp. 129–143, Anderson, R.S. (ed.). Pergamon Press, Oxford.

Wills, J. (1991) Dietary hypersensitivity in cats. *In Practice*, **13**, 87–93.

# 3 / Nutritional Diseases

## Introduction

Nutritional diseases arise as a direct result of faults in dietary formulation and/or feeding practices, and may broadly be classified into one of two groups:

1 Conditions associated with undernutrition, e.g. specific vitamin or mineral deficiencies.

2 Conditions associated with overnutrition, e.g. hypervitaminosis or obesity.

Whilst the theoretical potential exists for many single nutrient deficiencies, in practice, as has been noted in Chapter 2, relatively few are likely to be observed with any frequency. An important point to be remembered is that signs associated with nutrient deficiency may be observed in animals that are being fed diets that are apparently nutritionally adequate on chemical analysis. In these cases, nutrients which are present in the diet are biologically unavailable to the animal. This poor bioavailability may be due to the chemical form of a nutrient in the diet, or due to interaction between nutrients within poorly-balanced diets. For example, phosphorus present in phytates in cereals is poorly available, and high levels of calcium in diets may interfere with absorption of other divalent cations such as zinc.

Whilst inadequate intake of nutrients (with the exception of those where demands are met by body synthesis) would be expected to be associated with ill health, excessive intake of some nutrients is also harmful to the individual. Thus, for each nutrient there exists a range of different intakes which are compatible with optimal health, and departure from this range may be associated with overt disease, or at least, with suboptimal health (Fig. 3.1). The size of this range depends upon the individual nutrient and the life stage of the particular animal. The degree to which an individual nutrient is toxic depends on a number of factors, including whether it is stored in the body, or whether intakes above immediate needs are excreted. For example, with water-soluble vitamins where excesses are excreted in urine, oral toxicity is unlikely to occur, whereas it is potentially much more of a problem with the fat-soluble vitamins which are stored in the body. As noted, life stage can also exert an effect on the range of acceptable intakes (or dietary levels) of a particular nutrient. For example, the preferred range for calcium in a diet for a growing puppy is narrower than that which would be acceptable for an adult dog.

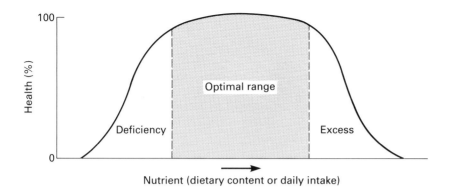

**Fig. 3.1** Nutrient intake and health. (After Kronfield & Banta, 1989. In *Nutrition of the Dog and Cat*, Burger, I.H. & Rivers, J.P.W. (eds). With the permission of Cambridge University Press.)

Problems of overnutrition related to specific nutrients are most likely to arise through injudicious supplementation of diets, or from poor raw material selection in home-prepared diets. Obesity, which is the most common form of overnutrition, and which is caused by excessive energy intake generally associated with incorrect feeding practices is discussed in Chapter 4.

Where nutritional diseases are suspected it may not always prove easy to identify the particular nutrient implicated, particularly as cases may be complicated by anorexia. Thus, a general approach to the dietary component of management that may be of value in many cases is to substitute a known nutritionally complete and balanced commercially-produced diet. This approach may often be simpler than trying to correct the levels of one or more nutrients in a suspect diet accurately. Indeed, it is likely that the wide availability of nutritionally-balanced commercial foods has led to a reduction in the incidence of many nutritional diseases. This chapter discusses a number of nutritional diseases that may still be observed on occasion.

## Hypervitaminosis A

Hypervitaminosis A results from prolonged, excessive intake of vitamin A. This may be due to overzealous dietary supplementation, for example with fish liver oils, or from poor dietary formulation using excessive quantities of foods rich in vitamin A. The condition has classically been associated with the feeding of large quantities of liver to cats, but cases have also been reported associated with feeding of certain fish (Petazzi *et al.*, 1989). β-carotene is not toxic in the same way as preformed vitamin A, as its hydrolysis and absorption from the gut are carefully regulated (Hayes,

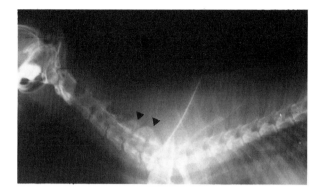

**Fig. 3.2** Skeletal changes (arrowed) associated with hypervitaminosis A in a cat. (Photograph by courtesy of A. Burnie.)

1982). Hypervitaminosis A is clinically important in cats, usually being observed in adults, although it has been reported in an adult dog and has been produced experimentally in growing kittens and dogs (Maddock *et al.*, 1949; Clark *et al.*, 1970a; Donoghue *et al.*, 1987).

A variety of clinical signs have been noted in cats fed high levels of vitamin A for several months. These include poor coat, lethargy, apprehension, reluctance to move, lameness and pain on neck palpation (Seawright *et al.*, 1967). Skeletal changes that occur are characterized by the development of multiple exostoses (Fig. 3.2). These are most noticeable on the cervical and thoracic vertebrae, where they may become confluent, and on the forelimbs. They occur around articular surfaces in the region of ligament and tendon attachment. In young animals shortening of longbones and damage to epiphyseal growth plates have been observed (Clark *et al.*, 1970a, b).

Evaluation of plasma vitamin A levels in experimental studies has indicated that although they tended to be higher in affected cats, there was overlap between affected and unaffected animals. Liver concentrations of vitamin A also tended to be higher in animals with skeletal disease, but again there was overlap with animals not showing skeletal changes (Seawright *et al.*, 1967).

Treatment of cats with hypervitaminosis A is essentially by dietary correction. Unfortunately, actually persuading a cat that has been fed large amounts of liver to change its diet may prove difficult, as this food is extremely palatable to cats. It may prove necessary to 'wean' the cat onto alternative foods gradually. Administration of lipotrophic substances such as methionine or choline has also been recommended (Whittick, 1974). Dietary change tends to bring about amelioration of clinical signs. However, skeletal changes persist, although substantial remodelling towards normal occurs with time. Damage to epiphyseal plates may be irreparable and long-bone growth permanently retarded (Bennett, 1976; Hayes, 1982).

## Hypervitaminosis D

Hypervitaminosis D is a relatively uncommon condition in dogs and cats. However, it has been reported as a result of injudicious dietary supplementation, or of rodenticide poisoning. The minimum lethal dose of calciferol in the dog is reported to be 4 mg/kg body weight, and cats may be more susceptible. However, as commercial preparations of this rodenticide usually contain only 0.1% of the active compound, quite large quantities would have to be eaten to induce acute toxicity (Burger & Flecknell, 1985). Hypervitaminosis D has also been produced in experimental studies.

Clinical signs reported from a series of four cases of hypervitaminosis D included gastro-intestinal disturbances, anorexia and polyuria/polydipsia (Pagès & Trouillet, 1984). Hypercalcaemia is characteristic of hypervitaminosis D, and although hyperphosphataemia was also noted in the clinical cases considered above, it was absent in an experimental study (Spangler et al., 1979). The development of renal pathology is associated with hypervitaminosis D, and metastatic calcification has been observed in the heart, lung, kidney and stomach in experimental studies (Mulligan & Strickler, 1948; Spangler et al., 1979). Renal insufficiency eventually led to the euthanasia of two of the cases mentioned above.

Successful treatment for hypercalcaemia, believed to be caused by rodenticide ingestion, included intravenous (IV) administration of 0.9% sodium chloride solution, initially at approximately twice maintenance levels, frusemide IV, prednisolone subcutaneously (SC), and calcitonin SC. Potassium chloride supplementation was given as needed throughout the period of fluid therapy to offset urinary losses. It was noted that treatment had to be continued for a prolonged period, and calcium levels closely monitored when it was withdrawn. It was also considered that the calcitonin could be a cause of anorexia (Fooshee & Forrester, 1990).

## Overnutrition and skeletal disease

The experiments reported by Hedhammer et al. (1974) showed that overnutrition of young, growing puppies of giant breeds could result in accelerated growth, and a variety of skeletal abnormalities including hypertrophic osteodystrophy, osteochondrosis dissecans and 'wobbler' syndrome. In this study there was excessive intake of a food rich in protein, energy, calcium and phosphorus, and thus it was not clear whether a single, or a combination, of dietary factors were primarily responsible for the problems observed. Subsequent studies in which just the calcium content of the diet was increased (to 3.3% on dry matter), indicated that excess intake of this mineral alone could be associated with skeletal changes leading to osteochondrosis, retained cartilage cone, radius curvus syndrome and stunted growth (Hazewinkel *et al.*, 1985).

Based on this evidence it is advisable that careful attention should be paid to both dietary composition and feeding level in growing puppies of the giant breeds. It appears undesirable to feed for a maximum rate of growth in these breeds.

## Calcium deficiency

The relationship between calcium and phosphorus, as has been noted in the previous chapter, requires not only that they are present in adequate amounts in the diet, but also in the correct ratio. A number of skeletal diseases may be associated with incorrect calcium and/or phosphorus levels and ratios in diets, of which the most common is probably nutritional secondary hyperparathyroidism. The basic underlying mechanism in this disease is a calcium deficiency resulting in a transient hypocalcaemia, stimulating the release of parathyroid hormone from the parathyroid glands (Bennett, 1976). The classic cause of this is feeding incorrectly balanced diets based on fresh meats. These are very poor sources of calcium, and have an adverse calcium:phosphorus ratio, for example, lean beef provides approximately 23 mg of calcium and 585 mg of phosphorus per 400 kcal (1.7 MJ) ME.

Excess phosphorus intake can also produce hypocalcaemia and hence parathyroid stimulation, even if dietary calcium is adequate, because of the interrelationship of calcium and phosphorus ions in solution (Krook *et al.*, 1963). Parathyroid hormone acts to help restore blood calcium through its effects on the kidney, decreasing calcium and increasing phosphorus excretion, and on bone, increasing resorption with resultant widespread skeletal effects. The disease is primarily one of the young, fast-growing animals and is particularly important clinically in the dog, although it has also been reported in cats.

A variety of clinical signs may be exhibited by affected animals, including lameness, abnormal gait or stance due to laxity of joint ligaments or tendons, inability or reluctance to stand or walk, and widespread bone pain. Severely affected animals may cry with pain in anticipation of being forced to move. Pathological fractures may occur in the longbones, particularly in the puppy, whereas in the cat the vertebral column appears more vulnerable. Fractures of the vertebrae may be associated with paraplegia (Bennett, 1976; Campbell, 1980; Campbell & Griffiths, 1984).

Radiography reveals poor bone density, thin cortices in severe cases, and commonly, pathological fractures. Growth plates generally appear normal,

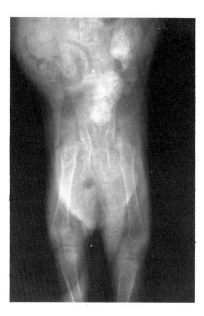

**Fig. 3.3** Nutritional secondary hyperparathyroidism in a cat. (Photograph by courtesy of A. Burnie.)

and are often associated with a radiodense area of preferential mineralization in the adjacent metaphysis (Bennett, 1976; Campbell & Griffiths, 1984) (Fig. 3.3).

For treatment of the condition, feeding of the unbalanced diet should be stopped, and a nutritionally adequate and balanced diet meeting the calcium and phosphorus requirements of the animal substituted. The simplest approach is to use a commercially prepared food suitable for growth. Further calcium supplementation to achieve a calcium : phosphorus ratio of 2 : 1 has been recommended for severely affected animals during the healing phase, but this should revert to the normal ratio when healing is complete (Capen & Martin, 1983). Confinement of affected animals during healing is advisable to reduce the risk of pathological fractures. Analgesics may be given, but recovery from pain is usually rapid after dietary correction.

Prevention of the condition may be accomplished by provision of good dietary advice to the owners of puppies and kittens, and by the use of good quality commercially prepared kitten and puppy foods.

## Vitamin D deficiency

The condition that has classically been associated with vitamin D deficiency is rickets, osteomalacia being the term given to the same condition in adults, however, uncertainty exists over the relative importance of vitamin

D and the dietary levels of calcium and phosphorus. Experimental studies have shown that rickets, complicated by osteoporosis, occurred in puppies that were fed diets deficient in calcium, phosphorus and vitamin D. Feeding the same diet with supplemental vitamin D largely prevented the rickets, but worsened the osteoporosis. Feeding the diet supplemented with adequate calcium and phosphorus, but without supplemental vitamin D, prevented skeletal disease. The base diet itself was considered to contain only a trace of vitamin D (Campbell & Douglas, 1965). Thus the growing dog appeared largely independent of a dietary supply of vitamin D, provided that the mineral content of the diet was adequate. However, more recent studies have shown that rickets can develop in dogs fed a diet deficient in vitamin D, but with normal calcium and phosphorus levels and ratio. In this study low plasma phosphate was noted in the dogs, presumably as a result of the hypovitaminosis D. This experiment also indicated that exposure to UV light could not prevent the development of rickets in dogs (Hazewinkel *et al.*, 1987).

Experimental studies in kittens have suggested that rickets may be produced with normal calcium and phosphorus levels and ratio (Gershoff *et al.*, 1957a), although more recent studies found no signs of bone disease, except for slight slowing of the rate of epiphyseal closure, despite long periods of vitamin D deprivation (Rivers *et al.*, 1979).

This condition is characterized by failure of normal mineralization of newly formed osteoid tissue and, in the young animal, also of the

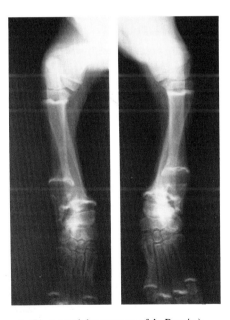

**Fig. 3.4** Rickets in a cat. (Photograph by courtesy of A. Burnie.)

cartilaginous matrix in the epiphyseal growth plates (Campbell & Griffiths, 1984). It is now considered to be a rare condition.

Clinical signs include lameness and inability to walk, lordosis, abnormal eruption of teeth and development of a plantigrade stance. Deformation of the bones may be noted, with bending of the shaft of longbones and enlargement at the epiphysis and metaphysis. Radiographically, widening of the epiphyseal growth plates is considered pathognomonic of the disease. Bone density throughout the skeleton is also reduced (Bennett 1976; Campbell & Griffiths, 1984) (Fig. 3.4). Hypocalcaemic tetany has also been reported in association with rickets in puppies (Lavelle, 1987).

Treatment is by dietary correction, ensuring that the substituted diet contains adequate vitamin D and minerals, the latter also in correct ratio. Given the above discussion on aetiology and the risks of hypervitaminosis D, substituting an adequate diet is probably preferable to trying to supplement the current diet with individual nutrients. An exception to this general advice would be in cases where an inborn error in vitamin D metabolism was suspected. Management of such a case using calcium supplementation and dihydrotachysterol has been reported (Johnson *et al.*, 1988).

## Vitamin A deficiency

Hypovitaminosis A is seldom reported clinically in the dog and cat, although a number of experimental studies have been conducted on the condition. It is worth reiterating the difference between the cat and the dog with regard to vitamin A sources, in that the cat is dependent on pre-formed (i.e. animal-derived) vitamin A, whereas the dog can utilize β-carotene.

The clinical signs that have been noted in deficiency in the dog include weight loss, anorexia, ataxia, xerophthalmia, conjunctivitis, corneal opacity and ulceration, skin lesions, metaplasia of bronchiolar epithelium, pneumonitis, increased susceptibility to infection, and in young dogs, faulty bone remodelling (National Research Council, 1985). An experimental study in cats reported weight loss as the most constant sign, occurring more rapidly in younger than in older kittens on the deficient diet. Cats also developed a serosanguinous exudate about the eyelids and muscle weakness and incoordination, especially of the hind limbs. The characteristic change observed in this study was squamous metaplasia in the respiratory tract, conjunctiva, salivary glands and endometrium. Extensive infectious sequelae were also noted in the lung, and occasionally in conjunctiva and salivary glands. Hypoplasia of seminiferous tubules and focal atrophy of the skin were also noted, and some cats showed a focal dysplasia of pancreatic exocrine tissues. Retardation of bone growth was not noted in this study, but this may have reflected the age of the animals used (Gershoff *et al.*, 1957b).

In addition to dietary history and clinical signs, assessment of serum vitamin A status may be useful in the diagnosis of hypovitaminosis A, with levels below approximately 200 IU/100 ml in kittens giving cause for concern (Scott & Scott, 1964). Where hypovitaminosis A is suspected, the diet should be corrected or supplementation given, although as with vitamin D supplementation, care should be taken to avoid oversupplementation.

Successful treatment with vitamin A supplementation of a small number of cases of a vitamin A-responsive dermatosis in dogs, characterized by medically refractory seborrhoeic skin disease, has also been reported (Scott, 1986).

## Vitamin E deficiency

Probably the best known condition associated with vitamin E deficiency is 'yellow fat disease' or pansteatitis in cats. This occurs when high levels of polyunsaturated fatty acids are fed with low levels of vitamin E, leading to the deposition of ceroid pigment in adipose tissue with fat cell necrosis and subsequent inflammation (Gaskell et al., 1975). In early reports, the condition was associated with cats fed predominantly on red tuna, but cases have also been recorded in cats fed other fish in their diet (Munson et al., 1958; Griffiths et al., 1960; Gaskell et al., 1975).

The major clinical signs observed in cases of pansteatitis include anorexia, depression, pyrexia and general tenderness. Subcutaneous fat may be lumpy on palpation, particularly on the ventral abdomen. A leucocytosis with neutrophilia and shift to the left may be present (Griffiths et al., 1960; Gaskell et al., 1975).

Treatment consists of dietary correction although, as with cats used to liver, this may prove difficult in some cases, and administration of vitamin E (20–25 IU b.i.d.). Corticosteroids may also be of value in some cases (Gaskell et al., 1975).

Vitamin E deficiency does not appear to be an important clinical entity in the dog, although the condition has been produced in a number of experimental studies. Use of large oral doses of vitamin E have been suggested as an alternative treatment for primary canine acanthosis nigricans if glucocorticoids are contraindicated (Scott & Walton, 1985).

## Essential fatty acid deficiency

Essential fatty acid (EFA) deficiency has been recorded experimentally in the dog and cat, although its true clinical significance is difficult to assess. Rivers (1982) commented that it is difficult to induce EFA deficiency in the cat without prolonged feeding of carefully designed diets. Notwithstanding this, EFAs are of considerable current interest in veterinary medicine, but more for their possible therapeutic role in certain dermatoses, rather than from a consideration of true deficiency. Apart from dietary deficiencies, EFA deficiency could occur as a result of intestinal malabsorption, in hepatic disease and where there is impaired function of enzymes involved in EFA metabolism (Lloyd, 1989).

Wide-ranging signs of EFA deficiency have been reported in the cat and dog. The gross clinical picture includes reduced growth in young animals and emaciation in adults. The coat may be roughened or staring, and in the cat, a greasy coat has also been noted. A variety of problems associated with reproduction have been described in the cat, including irregular or absent oestrus, frequent resorptions, stillbirths and neonatal deaths; male cats may also refuse to mate. Pathological and histological changes include fatty infiltration and degeneration of the liver in cats, and hyperplasia and hyperkeratosis of the skin in cats and dogs (Rivers & Frankel, 1980). EFA deficiency may be managed by change to an adequate diet, or by supplementation. As noted in the previous chapter, linoleic acid is the only EFA for which a requirement has been established in the dog, but the cat also requires a source of arachidonic acid for certain functions, such as reproduction in the female (McDonald et al., 1984).

The use of nutritional supplements containing EFAs in the management of allergic disease in dogs has become a subject of considerable interest. In one study, treatment with a supplement containing eicosapentaenoic, γ-linolenic, linoleic and α-linolenic acids resulted in a 50% or greater reduction in the level of pruritus in 33 of 93 allergic dogs (Miller et al., 1989). Positive results have also been obtained in other studies using EFA supplements. In one of these studies using evening primrose oil, there was little effect on pruritus, although other criteria such as coat condition and oedema showed marked improvements (Lloyd & Thomsett, 1989).

## Thiamin deficiency

Thiamin deficiency is one example of a single nutrient deficiency that may be encountered in practice. Although the condition is generally considered to be one primarily affecting cats, it has been recorded in sledge dogs fed on an all-fish diet, when presumably it occurred as a result of thiaminase present in the fish, and in dogs fed on cooked fresh meat, when presumably it resulted from destruction of the thiamin by cooking (Houston & Hulland, 1988; Read et al., 1977).

The development of thiamin deficiency in the cat can be divided into three stages with characteristic signs (Everett, 1944):

1 *Induction stage*, gradual loss of appetite, usually beginning during the second week of feeding, with complete anorexia by the fourth week, although the cat still shows interest in food. Vomiting may also occur. Walking is

normal until the end of the third or fourth week when slight ataxia is often present in the hind limbs.

2  *Critical stage*, characterized by nervous signs. The onset of this stage is sudden. Abnormal posture, ataxia and pupil dilation were the most constant features, and ventroflexion of the head and convulsions were also common.

3  *Terminal stage*, the animal becomes progressively weaker and passes into this stage, where it is prostrate. Death follows within a day or two.

The course of thiamin deficiency in this study developed rapidly and ended with death in 30–40 days. Clinical signs observed in naturally occurring disease in the dog include anorexia, spastic paraparesis and tetraparesis, recumbency, convulsions, coma and death (Read *et al.*, 1977; Houston & Hulland, 1988).

Treatment by injection of thiamin will bring about rapid recovery if the disease has not progressed too far. In the terminal stage treatment is not successful, and cats treated in the late critical stage may show some impairment for several weeks (Everett, 1944). The diet of the animal should also be corrected.

## Zinc deficiency

Experimental studies of zinc deficiency have been reported in the dog (Robertson & Burns, 1963; Sanecki *et al.*, 1982; Meyer *et al.*, 1986), and in the cat (Kane *et al.*, 1981). Naturally-occurring disease appears not to have been reported in the cat, whereas there are a number of reports of zinc-responsive dermatoses in the dog. Dietary zinc requirements are influenced by a number of other dietary components. For example, calcium is known to have an important influence; indeed diets high in calcium and low in zinc have been used experimentally to induce zinc deficiency (Roberston & Burns, 1963). Other dietary components may also have an influence on zinc availability. Phytate, which is present in most diets in which the primary protein source is of plant origin, has been shown to reduce zinc availability, and copper, iron, cadmium and chromium may compete for intestinal absorption sites (Oberleas *et al.*, 1962; Kunkle, 1980; Thoday, 1989). These observations serve to underline the importance of ensuring relative balance between nutrients, as well as avoiding absolute deficiencies. Their clinical importance is reflected in the view of van den Broek and Thoday (1986), who considered that the cases they observed resulted from dietary imbalances rather than from absolute deficiency of zinc, although they also suggested that inherent defects of zinc absorption could have contributed to some cases.

Two clinical syndromes have been reported that respond to zinc supplementation in dogs (Kunkle, 1980). Syndrome I occurs primarily in the Siberian husky and Alaskan malamute. The clinical signs include

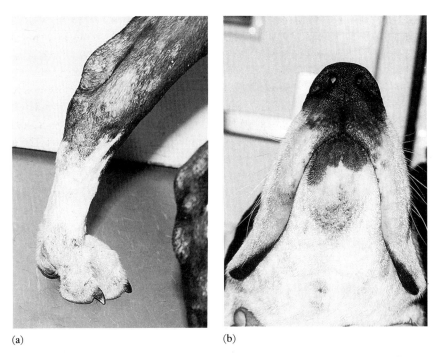

(a)                                            (b)

**Fig. 3.5** Lesions associated with zinc-responsive dermatosis. (Photograph by courtesy of
A. van den Broek.)

erythema, alopecia, scaling, crusting and suppuration around the mouth,
chin, eyes, ears and perineum (Fig. 3.5). Thick crusts may be present over
joints. Onset often occurs during puberty, although older dogs may sometimes be affected. Some dogs show lesions only when under stress (Kunkle,
1980; Degryse *et al.*, 1987). It seems likely that this syndrome arises from a
genetically-determined relative inability to absorb zinc, as is also seen in
chondrodysplasia in Alaskan malamutes (Brown *et al.*, 1978).

Many cases are reported as responding well to oral zinc supplementation, with 100 mg of zinc sulphate b.i.d. usually sufficient for huskies,
although more may be required in some cases. Therapy may need to be
continued indefinitely (Kunkle, 1980).

Syndrome II was reported in growing puppies fed diets containing high
levels of calcium. Severity of clinical signs, including dermatological ones,
was quite variable. Signs noted in puppies included the presence of hyper-
keratotic plaques over portions of the body, extreme thickening with fissur-
ing of the foot pads, and sometimes of the planum nasale. Some puppies
also seemed undersized, and some were anorexic and debilitated. Treatment
with zinc gave marked improvement, and continuation of supplementation
until adulthood was usually all that was necessary in these cases. It was also
noted that changing the diet alone could give the same improvement as
adding zinc (Kunkle, 1980).

Thoday (1989) suggested that there was considerable overlap in the character and distribution of the lesions of the two syndromes and that the essential difference was in the breeds and ages of the affected animals. He also reported seeing zinc-responsive dermatosis in numerous breeds with a wide age range. The factor common to most cases was the feeding of soya- or cereal-based diets in which it was suspected that zinc availability was reduced by interaction with other dietary factors. Important clinical signs included a dull, harsh coat with or without achromotrichia, erythema, seborrhoea sicca, bilaterally symmetrical white/yellow crusts affecting the head, limbs, scrotum and perineum, ceruminous otitis and peripheral lymphomegaly. Treatment was by oral zinc sulphate supplementation (10 mg/kg o.d. with food). Long-term management was by dietary change. It is likely that many of the types of diets implicated in these observations have now been modified to contain additional zinc, thus overcoming the problem of bioavailability, and resulting in a substantial reduction in the number of cases likely to be seen.

## Taurine deficiency

Taurine is an essential nutrient in the cat's diet, for the reasons discussed in Chapter 2. The association between lack of dietary taurine and retinal degeneration has been recognized for some time in the cat (Hayes et al., 1975), but more recently taurine deficiency has also been associated with other clinical conditions, including reproductive problems and dilated cardiomyopathy.

### Retinal degeneration

The ophthalmological changes in this condition have been described by Barnet and Burger (1980), and appear specific, at least in their early stages, to retinopathy from this cause. The first obvious visible changes occur in the area centralis, observed as a spot of increased reflectivity, which gradually increases in size, but remains clearly demarcated (Fig. 3.6). Lesions are usually bilaterally symmetrical. A dietary deficiency must be present for some months before changes appear. The lesions are progressive whilst the cat remains on a deficient diet, although visual defects are not apparent until the late stages of degeneration.

### Reproduction

Taurine deficiency has been shown to have marked effects on reproductive performance in breeding queens, and on growth and survival of their young. In one study, foetal resorption, abortion and stillbirth were observed

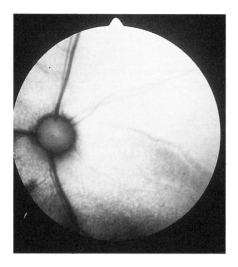

**Fig. 3.6** Taurine deficiency retinopathy in a cat.

in queens, with only 33% of pregnancies carried to term. Poor survivability and low birth weights were observed in kittens born alive. Poor growth and developmental abnormalities associated with cerebellar dysfunction occurred in surviving kittens (Sturman *et al.*, 1985, 1986).

### Dilated cardiomyopathy

Taurine deficiency has also been associated with dilated cardiomyopathy in cats (Pion *et al.*, 1987). Subsequent to this initial finding, it has now been reported that many cases of feline dilated cardiomyopathy are associated with low plasma taurine, and that administration of taurine to these cases can result in most showing an apparently permanent recovery of heart function. Taurine supplementation at a dose of 250 mg orally b.i.d. has been advised, in addition to standard therapy for dilated cardiomyopathy. Furthermore, it has been stated that the prognosis for cats surviving longer than 4 weeks after starting therapy can now be considered good to excellent (Pion *et al.*, 1988; Pion & Kittleson, 1990).

Taurine may be measured in whole blood or plasma. Whole blood provides the better assessment of body status, as plasma levels are influenced by dietary intake. The concentration of taurine in red blood cells is substantially higher than in plasma, therefore, if plasma is used care must be taken with sample collection to avoid haemolysis. Normal values for blood are in excess of 200 nmol/ml, and for plasma above 60 nmol/ml. The critical value below which a cat may be at risk of developing cardiomyopathy has been reported as approximately 20 nmol/ml in plasma (Pion & Kittleson, 1990). In the absence of measurements of plasma taurine, a review of the animal's diet may assist in predicting the likely taurine intake, remembering that sources of taurine are essentially limited to animal derived raw material.

Dietary correction and/or taurine supplementation may be given where taurine deficiency is suspected. Recommendations for the taurine content of prepared foods have been revised recently, as noted in the previous chapter. Data from a recent epidemiological survey is of interest in this regard; it was reported that the number of cases of feline dilated cardiomyopathy diagnosed at two referral practices decreased from 28% of feline echocardiographic diagnoses in 1986 to 6% in 1989. This change is presumably associated with the reformulation of cat foods following recognition of the problem of taurine availability (Skiles *et al.*, 1990).

# References

Barnet, K.C. & Burger, I.H. (1980) Taurine deficiency retinopathy in the cat. *Journal of Small Animal Practice*, **21**, 521–534.

Bennett, D. (1976) Nutrition and bone disease in the dog and cat. *Veterinary Record*, **98**, 313–320.

Brown, R.G., Hoag, G.N., Smart, M.E. & Mitchell, L.H. (1978) Alaskan malamute chondrodysplasia. V. Decreased gut zinc absorption. *Growth*, **42**, 1–6.

Burger, I.H. & Flecknell, P.A. (1985) Poisoning. In *Feline Medicine and Therapeutics*, pp. 321–338, Chandler, E.A., Gaskell, C.J. & Hilbery, A.D.R. (eds). Blackwell Scientific Publications, Oxford.

Campbell, J.R. (1980) Under-mineralisation in dogs and cats. In *Over and Undernutrition*, pp. 16–22, Edney, A.T.B. (ed.). Pedigree Petfoods, Melton Mowbray.

Campbell, J.R. & Douglas, T.A. (1965) The effect of low calcium intake and vitamin D supplements on bone structure in young growing dogs. *British Journal of Nutrition*, **19**, 339–351.

Campbell, J.R. & Griffiths, I.R. (1984) Bones and muscles. In *Canine Medicine and Therapeutics*, pp. 138–166, Chandler, E.A., Sutton, J.B. & Thompson, D.J. (eds). Blackwell Scientific Publications, Oxford.

Capen, C.C. & Martin, S.L. (1983) Calcium-regulating hormones and diseases of the parathyroid glands. In *Veterinary Internal Medicine*, pp. 1550–1591, Ettinger, S.J. (ed.). W.B. Saunders, Philadelphia.

Clark, L., Seawright, A.A. & Gartner, R.J.W. (1970a) Longbone abnormalities in kittens following vitamin A administration. *Journal of Comparative Pathology*, **80**, 113–121.

Clark, L., Seawright, A.A. & Hrdlicka, J. (1970b) Exostoses in hypervitaminotic A cats with optimal calcium–phosphorus intakes. *Journal of Small Animal Practice*, **11**, 553–561.

Degryse, A.-D., Fransen, J., Van Cutsem, J & Ooms, L. (1987) Recurrent zinc-responsive dermatosis in a Siberian husky. *Journal of Small Animal Practice*, **28**, 721–726.

Donoghue, S., Szanto, J. & Kronfeld, D.S. (1987) Hypervitaminosis A in a dog: an example of hospital dietetics. In *Nutrition, Malnutrition and Dietetics in the Dog and Cat*, pp. 94–96, Edney, A.T.B. (ed.). British Veterinary Association, London/ Waltham Centre for Pet Nutrition, Melton Mowbray.

Everett, G.M. (1944) Observations on the behaviour and neurophysiology of acute thiamin deficient cats. *American Journal of Physiology*, **141**, 439–448.

Fooshee, S.K. & Forrester, S.D. (1990) Hypercalcemia secondary to cholecalciferol rodenticide toxicosis in two dogs. *Journal of the American Veterinary Medical Association*, **196**, 1265–1268.

Gaskell, C.J., Leedale, A.H. & Douglas, S.W. (1975) Pansteatitis in the cat: a report of four cases. *Journal of Small Animal Practice*, **16**, 117–121.

Gershoff, S.N., Andrus, S.B., Hegsted, D.M. & Lentini, E.A. (1957b) Vitamin A deficiency in cats. *Laboratory Investigation*, **6**, 227–240.

Gershoff, S.N., Legg, M.A., O'Connor, F.J. & Hegsted, D.M. (1957a) The effect of vitamin D deficient diets containing various Ca:P ratios on cats. *Journal of Nutrition*, **63**, 79–93.

Griffiths, R.C., Thornton, G.W. & Willson, J.E. (1960) Pansteatitis ('yellow fat') in cats. *Journal of the American Veterinary Medical Association*, **137**, 126–128.

Hayes, K.C. (1982) Nutritional problems in cats: taurine deficiency and vitamin A excess. *Canadian Veterinary Journal*, **23**, 2–5.

Hayes, K.C., Carey, R.E. & Schmidt, S.Y. (1975) Retinal degeneration associated with taurine deficiency in the cat. *Science*, **188**, 949–951.

Hazewinkel, H.A.W., Goedegebuure, S.A., Poulos, P.W. & Wolvekamp, W.T.C. (1985) Influences of chronic calcium excess on the skeletal development of growing great Danes. *Journal of the American Animal Hospital Association*, **21**, 377–391.

Hazewinkel, H.A.W., How, K.L., Bosch, R., Goodegebuure, S.A. & Voorhout, G. (1987) Inadequate photosynthesis of vitamin D in dogs. In *Nutrition, Malnutrition and Dietetics of the Dog and Cat*, pp. 66–68, Edney, A.T.B. (ed.). British Veterinary Association, London/Waltham Centre for Pet Nutrition, Melton Mowbray.

Hedhammer, Å., Wu, F.-M., Krook, L., Schryver, H.F., De Lahunta, A., Whalen, J.P., Kallfelz, F.A., Nunez, E.A., Hintz, H.F., Sheffey, B.E. & Ryan, G.D. (1974) Overnutrition and skeletal disease. *Cornell Veterinarian*, **64**, Suppl. 5.

Housten, D.M. & Hulland, T.J. (1988) Thiamin deficiency in a team of sled dogs. *Canadian Veterinary Journal*, **29**, 383–384.

Johnson, K.A., Church, D.B., Barton, R.J. & Wood, A.K.W. (1988) Vitamin D dependent rickets in a Saint Bernard dog. *Journal of Small Animal Practice*, **29**, 657–666.

Kane, E., Morris, J.G., Rogers, Q.R., Ihrke, P.J. & Cupps, P.T. (1981) Zinc deficiency in the cat. *Journal of Nutrition*, **111**, 488–495.

Krook, L., Barrett, R.B., Usui, K. & Wolke, R.E. (1963) Nutritional secondary hyperparathyroidism in the cat. *Cornell Veterinarian*, **53**, 224–246.

Kunkle, G.A. (1980) Zinc responsive dermatoses in dogs. In *Current Veterinary Therapy VII. Small Animal Practice*, pp. 472–476, Kirk, R.W. (ed.). W.B. Saunders, Philadelphia.

Lavelle, R. (1987) Hypocalcaemic tetany associated with rickets in the dog. In *Nutrition, Malnutrition and Dietetics in the Dog and Cat*, pp. 101–103, Edney, A.T.B. (ed.). British Veterinary Association, London/Waltham Centre for Pet Nutrition, Melton Mowbray.

Lloyd, D.H. (1989) Essential fatty acids and skin disease. *Journal of Small Animal Paractice*, **30**, 207–212.

Lloyd, D.H. & Thomsett, L.R. (1989) Essential fatty acid supplementation in the treatment of canine atopy. *Veterinary Dermatology*, **1**, 41–44.

McDonald, M.L. Rogers, Q.R., Morris, J.G. & Cupps, P.T. (1984) Effect of linoleate and arachidonate deficiencies on reproduction and spermatogenesis in the cat. *Journal of Nutrition*, **114**, 719–726.

Maddock, C.L., Wolbach, S.B. & Maddock, S. (1949) Hypervitaminosis A in the dog. *Journal of Nutrition*, **39**, 117–137.

Meyer, H., Hommerich, G., Schoon, H.-A. & Mundt, C. (1986) Experimenteller Zinkmangel bei ausgewachsenen Hunden. *Kleintierpraxis*, **31**, 21–28.

Miller, W.H., Griffin, C.E., Scott, D.W., Angarano, D.K. & Norton A.L. (1989) Clinical trial of DVM Derm Caps in the treatment of allergic disease in dogs: a nonblinded study. *Journal of the American Animal Hospital Association*, **25**, 163–168.

Mulligan, R.M. & Strickler, F.L. (1948) Metastatic calcification produced in dogs by hypervitaminosis D and haliphagia. *American Journal of Pathology*, **24**, 451–466.

Munson, T.O., Holzworth, J., Small, E., Witzel, S., Jones, T.C. & Luginbühl, H. (1958) Steatitis ('yellow fat') in cats fed canned red tuna. *Journal of the American Veterinary Medical Association*, **133**, 563–568.

National Research Council (1985) *Nutrient Requirements of Dogs*. National Academy Press, Washington, DC.

Oberleas, D., Muhrer, M.E. & O'Dell, B.L. (1962) Effect of phytic acid on zinc availability and parakeratosis in swine. *Journal of Animal Science*, **21**, 57–61.

Pagès, J.-P. & Trouillett, J.-L. (1984) Néphropathie hypercalcémique: a propos de quatre intoxications argus par la vitamine D chez le chien. *Practique Medicale et Chirugicale de l'Animal de Compagne*, **19**, 293–300.

Petazzi, F., Crovace, A. & Di Bello, A. (1989) Alterazioni scheletriche da ipervitaminosi A nel gatto. *Obiettivi – E – Documenti Veterinari*, **10**, 79–83.

Pion, P.D. & Kittleson, M.D. (1990) Taurine's role in clinical practice. *Journal of Small Animal Practice*, **31**, 510–518.

Pion, P.D., Kittleson, M.D., Delellis, L.A., Newhouse, C.A. & Rogers, Q.R. (1988) Recovery of myocardial function in cats with dilated cardiomyopathy secondary to taurine deficiency: one year followup (Abstract). *Circulation*, **78** (Suppl.), 340.

Pion, P.D., Kittleson, M.D., Rogers, Q.R. & Morris, J.G. (1987) Myocardial failure in cats associated with low plasma taurine: a reversible cardiomyopathy. *Science*, **237**, 764–768.

Read, D.H., Jolly, R.D. & Alley, M.R. (1977) Polioencephalomalacia of dogs with thiamin deficiency. *Veterinary Pathology*, **14**, 103–112.

Rivers, J.P.W. (1982) Essential fatty acids in cats. *Journal of Small Animal Practice*, **23**, 563–576.

Rivers, J.P.W. & Frankel, J.L. (1980) Fat in the diet of dogs and cats. In *Nutrition of the Dog and Cat*, pp. 67–100, Anderson, R.S. (ed.). Pergamon Press, Oxford.

Roberston, B.T. & Burns, M.J. (1963) Zinc metabolism and the zinc deficiency syndrome in the dog. *American Journal of Veterinary Research*, **24**, 997–1002.

Sanecki, R.K., Corbin, J.E. & Forbes, R.M. (1982) Tissue changes in dogs fed a zinc deficient ration. *American Journal of Veterinary Research*, **43**, 1642–1646.

Scott, D.W. (1986) Vitamin A-responsive dermatosis in the cocker spaniel. *Journal of the American Animal Hospital Association*, **22**, 125–129.

Scott, D.W. & Walton, D.K. (1985) Clinical evaluation of oral vitamin E for the treatment of primary canine acanthosis nigricans. *Journal of the American Animal Hospital Association*, **21**, 345–350.

Scott, P.P. & Scott, M.G. (1964) Vitamin A and reproduction in the cat. *Journal of Reproduction and Fertility*, **8**, 270.

Seawright, A.A., English, P.B. & Gartner, R.J.W. (1967) Hypervitamiosis A and deforming cervical spondylosis of the cat. *Journal of Comparative Pathology*, **77**, 29–39.

Skiles, M.L., Pion, P.D., Hird, D.W., Kittleson, M.D., Stein, B.S., Lewis, J. & Peterson, M.D. (1990) Epidemiologic evaluation of taurine deficiency and dilated cardiomyopathy in cats (Abstract). *Journal of Veterinary Internal Medicine*, **4**, 117.

Spangler, W.L., Gribble, D.H. & Lee, T.C. (1979) Vitamin D intoxication and the pathogenesis of vitamin D nephropathy in the dog. *American Journal of Veterinary Research*, **40**, 73–83.

Sturman, J.A., Gargano, A.D., Messing, J.M. & Imaki, H. (1986) Feline maternal taurine deficiency: effect on mother and offspring. *Journal of Nutrition*, **116**, 655–667.

Sturman, J.A., Moretz, R.C., French, J.H. & Wisniewski, H.M. (1985) Taurine deficiency in the developing cat: persistence of the cerebellar external granule cell layer. *Journal of Neuroscience Research*, **13**, 405–416.

Thoday, K.L. (1989) Diet related zinc-responsive skin disease in dogs: a dying dermatosis? *Journal of Small Animal Practice*, **30**, 213–215.

Van den Broek, A.H.M. & Thoday, K.L. (1986) Skin disease in dogs associated with zinc deficiency: a report of five cases. *Journal of Small Animal Practice*, **27**, 313–323.

Whittick, W.G. (1974) Metabolic bone diseases. In *Canine Orthopaedics*, pp. 39–54, Lea & Febiger, Philadelphia.

# 4 / Dietary Management of Clinical Diseases

## Introduction

There is a growing awareness that in many cases successful therapy relies not only on the use of drugs but also on supplying an appropriate form of nutrition. Indeed the patient may respond and subsequently recover more rapidly when consideration is given to diet and not drugs alone. In some conditions diet may be the major component of therapy, such as in gluten sensitivity, while in others it helps to spare an organ from additional workload, such as in hepatic or renal disease.

The types of diet required in the management of clinical disease vary considerably. The recognition of these varied dietary requirements has resulted in a large number of veterinary diets becoming available to practitioners, thereby making dietary management much easier for the clinician and the client alike. Home-made diets are not only time consuming in their preparation but often fail to provide uniformity of composition from day to day.

It is important to emphasize that if the patient will not eat the appropriate veterinary diet for the clinical condition present, another form of nutrition must be provided. It is preferable to provide a less than ideal protein calorie support than to allow the animal to starve. This is because starvation creates a negative nitrogen and energy balance with loss of lean muscle mass and increased nitrogen waste disposal.

The intention of this chapter is to discuss the role of nutrition in the treatment of a wide range of clinical conditions. In some cases diet plays a minor role in the regimes which are used, while in others it plays a major part in the therapeutic strategy.

## Gastro-intestinal disorders

### Vomiting

The dog has a highly developed vomiting centre and may vomit at will. The extensive aetiology of vomiting includes emotion, excitement, vestibular disease, visceral inflammation, toxaemic states and the influence of some drugs. As there are many non-gastric causes for vomiting, it is important to determine the underlying cause if treatment is to be successful.

Acute gastritis is the most common cause of vomiting especially in the dog. This is often associated with dietary indiscretions which are more rarely observed in cats due to their fastidious eating habits. Although acute gastritis can occur on its own, it is more often associated with concurrent enteritis.

Normally when food enters the stomach the fundus relaxes to accommodate it without increasing intragastric pressure (receptive relaxation). The antrum and pylorus are involved in grinding the solid food into a homogenate before release into the duodenum. Food leaves the stomach in an orderly sequence starting with fluids, then carbohydrate and protein, while fats and fibre leave the stomach last (Hinder & Kelly, 1977; Twedt, 1983; Hall et al., 1988).

When acute gastritis is present, receptive relaxation fails and intragastric pressure increases to a point where vomition occurs. The antral grinder may also fail, so retaining food in the stomach. This will be vomited hours after feeding if the intragastric pressure is not too high. Food and fluid entering the stomach stimulate the release of acid and pepsin which may further inflame the gastric mucosa. It is for these reasons that total gastric rest is advocated in acute gastritis, allowing the inflamed mucosa a chance to heal.

Ringer's solution should be given IV to correct fluid and electrolyte losses in gastritis followed by physiological saline. If vomiting persists even when the stomach is left empty, an anti-emetic such as metoclopramide at 0.5–1 mg/kg 8-hourly, may be useful in reducing the vomition which is weakening to the animal and results in further fluid and electrolyte loss. Cimetidine reduces acid production which may be useful in preventing further inflammation to the gastric mucosa.

When vomiting has stopped for at least 24 hours, small amounts of oral rehydrant may be offered, if vomiting does not recur, oral rehydrants may be continued in place of IV fluid therapy. Subsequently offer half the normal daily requirement of a highly-digestible, low-fat (<6% DM) (dry matter) diet in two or three meals per day. Chicken, fish, scrambled egg, rabbit and boiled rice would be suitable, or a commercial low-fat veterinary diet may be used. By using a low-fat, low-fibre (<2% DM) diet the food will pass out of the stomach more rapidly (Table 4.1). This is important in order to minimize intragastric pressure and to avoid compromising already suspect antral mixing.

The diet described above should be fed for 3 or 4 days and if vomiting does not recur a slow return to normal feeding should be permitted over a further 3 days.

Cases of chronic gastritis require to be investigated and classified following gastric biopsy collection, but generally benefit from a similar highly-digestible low-fat, low-fibre diet. However, these cases will require specific drug therapy in addition to diet in order to obtain a satisfactory resolution.

**Table 4.1** A summary of dietary requirements which may be of value in patients with gastro-intestinal disease. (DM = dry matter)

| Condition | Dietary management |
|---|---|
| Vomiting | Initially nil by mouth; once vomiting stops oral rehydrants, then highly digestible low-fat (<6% DM) low-fibre (<2% DM) diet; slow return to a suitable 'normal' diet |
| GDV | Feed a moist diet b.i.d., avoid cereal-based diet; highly-digestible high-energy dense diets so volume ingested is small |
| Diarrhoea | Dietary rest for 24 hours; highly-digestible, low-fat (<6% DM), low-fibre (<2% DM) diet with increased vitamin content; feed diet as two or three small meals/day |
| Diet sensitivity | Single/limited protein source, gluten-free; highly-digestible, hypoallergenic or elimination diets |
| Malabsorption | As for diarrhoea; possibly MCTs at 1–2 ml/kg o.d. |
| Coprophagia | Check for possible disease causing coprophagia; high-energy dense diet, occasionally better on high-fibre (>10% DM) diets |
| Constipation | High-fibre (>10% DM) diet; or add bulking agent to diet such as sterculia, ispaghula, bran |
| Colitis | |
|   Acute | As for diarrhoea |
|   Chronic | Single/limited protein source, highly-digestible, low-fibre (<2% DM) diet |
| Flatulence | Highly-digestible low-fat (<6% DM), low-fibre (<2% DM) diet; avoid soya, milk, vegetables |

## Gastric dilatation and volvulus

The aetiology of gastric dilatation and volvulus (GDV) is not understood but the following factors have been implicated: exercise and excitement after feeding, use of cereal-based diets, overdistension of the stomach, aerophagia, breed predisposition (great Danes, boxers, Weimaraners, bassets, Dobermanns, Irish setters, German shepherds), gastric stasis, gastric motility disorders, and lax gastric ligaments (Simpson & Else, 1991a). Clinically the signs of GDV are well recognized and diagnosis may be made following lateral radiography, passage of a stomach tube and/or exploratory laparotomy.

As the aetiology is not clearly understood, advice regarding dietary management is difficult. Dry cereal-based diets do not adversely affect gastric motility, as previously thought (Burrows *et al.*, 1985), but Van Kruiningen *et al.* (1987) suggested that cereal-based diets may nonetheless predispose to GDV by creating a larger stomach capacity and delayed gastric emptying due to overdistension. Leib and Martin (1987) did not find any association between type of diet and the development of GDV. It is generally thought that gas accumulation is not a consequence of bacterial fermentation as there is very little hydrogen or methane present. However carbon dioxide levels are often elevated and it has been suggested that this occurs when bicarbonate in saliva reacts with $H^+$ ions from gastric acid (Caywood et al., 1977). Aerophagia has also been suggested as a cause of gastric gas accumulation. Although bacterial numbers are usually low in the empty stomach they may increase after feeding when fermentation of food may occur. *Clostridia* spp. have been detected in GDV cases (Van Kruiningen et al., 1974), but were not found in another study (Caywood et al., 1977). It has been suggested that failure to eructate may be the reason for gas accumulation (Strombeck & Guilford, 1990a). Anatomical problems associated with the gastro-oeosphageal high pressure zone may be important in this respect.

GDV presents as an emergency requiring immediate fluid therapy and relief of gastric distension and shock. Following this the stomach position should be corrected surgically. Prevention of further episodes of GDV is achieved by gastropexy in most cases, and dietary management.

Until the aetiology of GDV is better understood it is difficult to give precise advice regarding dietary management. However the following dietary advice may be of value: avoid exercise and excitement prior to and following feeding, divide the daily ration into two meals to prevent overdistension of the stomach, never allow the dog to feed ad lib or ingest large amounts of water, use a moist meat-based diet rather than a dry cereal-based diet, a low fat diet which is also highly digestible will encourage rapid gastric emptying. Alternatively, feeding a high-calorie dense diet will reduce the volume of food provided and so may reduce the risk of GDV (see Table 4.1).

## Diarrhoea

Diarrhoea is the clinical manifestation of an intestinal disturbance which results in an increased volume or fluid content of the faeces. Normal faeces contain approximately 70% water but in diarrhoea the water content may be greater than 85% (Markwell, 1988). Diarrhoea is usually classified according to the mechanism which is involved into the following groups: osmotic diarrhoea, increased permeability, secretory diarrhoea, or motility diarrhoea.

Osmotic diarrhoea is associated with retention of nutrients within the intestine due to a failure in either digestion or absorption. The retained nutrients exert an osmotic force which retains fluid within the intestinal lumen resulting in diarrhoea. Conditions associated with osmotic diarrhoea include: exocrine pancreatic insufficiency (EPI), small intestinal disease, and viral infections which cause villus atrophy. Classically the diarrhoea stops when the patient is fasted.

The intestine is normally permeable proximally to allow fluid to enter the lumen to assist in digestion and absorption. However permeability decreases further along the intestine and is normally absent in the ileum and colon. Severe inflammation of the intestine and cardiac disease, which increases intestinal hydrostatic pressure, may induce a marked increase in porosity. Where this becomes advanced, plasma protein can escape into the intestinal lumen creating a protein-losing enteropathy.

Secretory diarrhoea occurs when the cells at the base of the intestinal villi, in the crypts of Leiberkühn, increase their secretion. When secretion becomes greater than net absorption, diarrhoea develops. Various agents are known to switch on intestinal secretion, including cholera toxin and toxins from *Escherichia coli* and *Salmonella* spp. Bacterial degradation of bile acids and dietary fat produces two further chemicals which can switch on secretion: deconjugated bile acids and hydroxy fatty acids.

It is generally thought that diarrhoea is associated with increased intestinal motility. In fact the reverse is usually more accurate. In most cases there is a loss in segmentation which is the motility pattern associated with mixing the intestinal contents and aiding absorption. Peristalsis, however, is normally retained and as there is an increased volume of intestinal contents this may give the impression of hypermotility.

Acute enteritis is common in the dog due to its depraved eating habits while it is much less often observed in cats. Where such a mechanism is implicated in the aetiology, the patient will normally respond well to symptomatic therapy without recourse to a clinical investigation. However, where chronic diarrhoea is present, that is diarrhoea which has been present for more than 3 weeks and which is unresponsive to treatment, a full clinical investigation will be required to obtain a definitive diagnosis. This is essential in order to establish a specific treatment regime (see EPI, malabsorption, dietary sensitivity).

The commonest cause of diarrhoea in dogs is dietary indiscretion such as overeating, consumption of soiled foods or sudden dietary change. Where there is no associated vomiting present oral rehydrants may be used, but otherwise dietary rest for 24–48 hours will be enough to produce a remission. At this time a diet may be offered which is low in fat (<6% DM) and fibre (<2% DM) (see Table 4.1). A low fat component is important to minimize the production of hydroxy fatty acids which would stimulate further secretion. Diets with this composition include chicken, fish, cooked eggs or cottage cheese with boiled rice. Alternatively a suitable veterinary diet may be fed. In all cases the diet should be offered in small, frequent meals each day and, assuming no recurrence of diarrhoea, slowly returned to normal over the subsequent week. Time should be spent discussing normal dietary management with the client to ensure similar problems do not occur in the future.

Antibiotics should not be used in the majority of diarrhoeas as they are of little therapeutic value and may induce gut flora problems resulting in chronic diarrhoea. Of much greater value are motility modifiers which restore segmentation, such as loperamide at 0.08 mg/kg b.i.d. in dogs and cats or diphenoxylate at 0.05–0.1 mg/kg 8-hourly for dogs (Strombeck & Guilford, 1990b).

Some foods should always be avoided in animals which are predisposed to diarrhoea. Milk contains large amounts of lactose and some adult dogs may lack adequate levels of lactase, the brush border enzyme required to digest this disaccharide (see Chapter 2). Raw eggs contain a trypsin inhibitor which is destroyed by cooking (Murdoch, 1986). Egg protein has a high biological value and is very useful in enteric disturbances so long as it is cooked first.

## Dietary sensitivity

In veterinary medicine it is customary to use the terms food allergy or hypersensitivity for any abnormal reaction to food irrespective of the aetiology (Wills, 1991). The vast majority of pets ingest food and do not become sensitized, but in a small number of cases immunological mechanisms become activated against specific antigens. Antigens are almost always proteins, especially glycoproteins which are often resistant to digestion and heat, thus maintaining their antigenicity (Strombeck & Guilford, 1990b). Milk protein, soya bean, wheat, beef, egg, horse meat, chicken, pork and yeast have all been incriminated in dogs (August, 1985; White, 1986). In cats the list of apparent food allergens is very similar but may also include fish (Wills, 1991).

Clinically the reaction may occur suddenly after months or years on the food concerned and the reactions are not seasonal. There is no breed, age or sex predisposition. Dermatological signs are most frequently observed and include pruritus, urticaria, otitis externa and miliary dermatitis in cats (Carlotti et al., 1990). Gastro-intestinal signs may occur on their own or together with skin changes. Vomiting and diarrhoea (with or without blood) are most frequently reported (Dakin, 1988), while lymphocytic–plasmacytic colitis has been recorded (Nelson et al., 1984). Occasionally a circulating eosinophilia is observed.

Gluten sensitivity is a specific and well-documented form of food hypersensitivity which has been observed in the Irish setter (Hall & Batt, 1988). In this specific case there is a familial tendency to the condition. It is thought to occur because of increased permeability of the intestine, allowing the antigen to evoke a delayed hypersensitivity reaction.

Treatment of food sensitivity involves removal of the antigen from the diet if this can be identified. In the case of gluten sensitivity it is necessary to offer a veterinary or other diet known to be gluten free for the rest of the dog's life (see Table 4.1). The intestinal changes are reversible and normal intestinal function returns within 6 weeks of dietary correction. In many cases the antigen is not identified and an elimination diet must be fed using a diet with a single or limited protein sources, ideally one(s) to which the pet has not previously been exposed (Markwell, 1988). Even when the diet is free of the sensitizing antigen, clinical signs may take several weeks to disappear.

When the patient is stabilized, single foods may be added to the regime in order to determine foods which can be tolerated and to identify the possible antigen. Normally, clinical signs will recur within 7 days of feeding the antigen. Each orginal food should be fed in turn until all the diet has been provocatively tested. In many cases in the author's experience the client will opt to continue feeding a hypoallergenic veterinary diet for the remainder of the animal's life.

**Malabsorption**

There are several conditions which may result in small intestinal malabsorption in dogs and cats. These include lymphocytic–plasmacytic enteritis, eosinophilic enteritis, regional enteritis, villus atrophy and lymphosarcoma. The aetiology of these conditions is still poorly understood although parasites, dietary sensitivities and immune reactions to viruses or bacterial toxins may be implicated. Diagnosis involves the evaluation of blood chemistry, absorption tests and intestinal biopsy.

Protein-losing enteropathy may be considered as an end stage disease involving any of the above conditions when present in an advanced stage. Lymphangiectasia is a specific protein-losing enteropathy involving obstruction of lymphatic drainage from the intestine. Intestinal permeability reaches a point where plasma proteins may leak into the intestinal lumen. Diagnosis is based on the tests for malabsorption together with detection of a panhypoproteinaemia and assessment of intestinal permeability.

Treatment of malabsorption usually involves drug and dietary therapy. Prednisolone is given to reduce the immune response and infiltration of the intestine with inflammatory cells. The drug also has a direct effect on the enterocytes, improving their absorptive capacity. Concurrent bacterial overgrowth can be treated with tylosin (Simpson & Else, 1991b). Dietary management usually involves the use of a veterinary diet containing limited protein sources to which ideally the patient has not been previously exposed. As enterocyte function is disturbed it is advisable to use a low-fat (<6% DM), low-fibre (<2% DM) diet based on a highly-digestible, carbohydrate-rich energy source such as rice (see Table 4.1). Increased levels of vitamins should also be incorporated within the diet. Vitamin K deficiency has been recorded in cats with intestinal malabsorption (Edwards & Russell, 1987), and B vitamin deficiency may occur with prolonged anorexia and diarrhoea (Buffington, 1986). In addition, folate levels may also fall in malabsorptive states (Strombeck & Guilford, 1990c).

Where lymphangiectasia has been diagnosed, a low-fat (<6% DM and ideally <4% DM) diet is of particular importance, due to the loss of lacteal function (Burns, 1982). These patients will depend on carbohydrate for energy, although medium chain triglyceride (MCT) may be included in the diet to supplement the energy levels (1–2 ml/kg/day). The route of absorption for MCT differs from normal dietary fat as it is mostly absorbed into the portal vein and not the lacteal. Enteric lymphosarcoma is rarely treated and carries a very guarded prognosis.

**Coprophagia**

This is a problem which is more commonly observed in dogs than cats. It is an unpleasant habit which is usually due to a depraved appetite or pica, but may be associated with an underlying disease process or a deficiency. It is not uncommon for dogs to eat rabbit, sheep or horse faeces, but where they eat their own faeces a careful clinical examination should be carried out to determine if there is an underlying cause.

Where the problem is thought to be habitual then it should be ensured that the garden is kept clear of faeces. A highly-digestible low-residue diet which has a high energy density should be fed. Occasionally a high-fibre diet may be more effective although the reason is not clear (see Table 4.1). In individual cases the clinician may have to try several diets before finding one which is suitable.

In situations where an underlying cause is thought to be present or where the dog fails to respond to one of the above regimes, an investigation should be carried out. In the author's experience EPI is the most common clinical cause of coprophagia in dogs.

**Constipation**

This may be defined as an inability to pass, or a difficulty in passing, faeces. There is a consequent retention of faecal material in the rectum and colon. The longer this occurs the more water will be resorbed from the faeces and the harder they will become. Impaction will occur and the animal will be physically unable to defaecate.

The aetiology of constipation is extensive and includes:
1 Dietary factors such as feeding bones, hunting cats which ingest hair and fur, and where there is inadequate water intake.
2 Pain associated with the colon, rectum, anus or anal glands, or to orthopaedic conditions preventing correct posturing.

**3** Obstruction to the passage of faeces following prostatic hyperplasia, tumours, rectal/anal strictures or extracolonic masses.

**4** Neurological problems of which the most frequent are intervertebral disc lesions.

**5** Drugs such as barium sulphate, sucralfate, antacids, codeine and diuretics.

**6** Lack of exercise and hospitalization (Sherding, 1990).

Clinical signs associated with constipation include dyschesia, tenesmus and haematochesia. Eventually anorexia, depression and vomiting occur, together with abdominal discomfort and arching of the back.

Initial treatment will involve the manual removal of impacted faeces from the colon and rectum. However once this has been achieved it will be necessary to prevent further recurrence of the constipation. This is best achieved by correction of the underlying cause together with dietary management.

The ingestion of bones should be prevented and adequate exercise should be provided. A diet should be fed which provides a soft but formed stool and encourages regular evacuation of the bowel. Most commercial pet diets are low in crude fibre (<4% DM) and are of little value in preventing constipation. Low dietary fibre and thus low-residue diets are contraindicated for the management of these cases, as they do not adequately stimulate colonic peristalsis. Therefore, a high-fibre (>10% DM) diet should be fed (Hoskins, 1990), such as one of the commercial veterinary diets or an ordinary diet supplemented with bran (1 tablespoonful/400 g tinned food), or another bulk forming agent (Burrows, 1986), such as sterculia or ispaghula husk (see Table 4.1). The patient should be allowed access to the garden within 30 minutes after feeding to further stimulate defaecation.

**Colitis**

This is a condition which is being detected with increasing frequency in dogs and is seen to a lesser extent in the cat. Several forms of colitis have been documented including parasitic colitis, eosinophilic colitis, histiocytic colitis, granulomatous colitis and lymphocytic–plasmacytic colitis (Simpson & Else, 1991c). Histiocytic colitis is rare and has only been reported in boxers, French bulldogs and cats (Kennedy & Cello, 1966; Van der Gaag *et al.*, 1978; Van Kruiningen & Dobbin, 1979). Lymphocytic–plasmacytic colitis is the form most commonly detected in the UK and it appears to have a multiple aetiology, although dietary sensitivity may be important. There appears to be no breed, age or sex predisposition to colitis in the dog or cat.

Clinically animals present with a history of chronic intractable diarrhoea which is usually small in volume and passed frequently; it often contains blood and/or mucus. Urgency, tenesmus, dyschesia and vomiting are additional clinical signs in some cases. Diagnosis is most easily obtained following endoscopic examination of the colon with biopsy collection and histological examination.

Treatment should involve removal of any underlying cause but traditionally involves the use of sulphasalazine therapy. Diet may be very important in the management of colitis, especially if dietary sensitivity is suspected. In acute exacerbations a highly-digestible, low-fat (<6% DM) diet is required so that small amounts of food residues reach the inflamed colon. This reduces distension and irritation, relieving the clinical signs (Zimmer, 1986). In chronic colitis several diets have been proposed. A high-fibre diet (>10% DM) designed to 'normalize' the colonic motility has been suggested. Mixed success has been obtained with this diet, probably because varying types of fibre have been used; the amount given and the form given have also varied. Recently, considerable interest has been shown in the possibility that a protein dietary sensitivity may be involved. Some success can be achieved using a single protein source such as chicken, lamb, fish or cottage cheese, or one of the commercial veterinary elimination diets (see Table 4.1). Success depends on the selection of the right protein, to which the animal has not been previously sensitized (Nelson et al., 1984; Simpson & Else, 1991c). It has been suggested that dry, cereal-based diets should be avoided (Burrows, 1988).

## Flatulence

The aetiology of this common anti-social problem is not known. Gas is normally produced in the intestine of dogs and cats, but the level and type of gas can vary considerably. Air may enter the gastro-intestinal tract following aerophagia, or gas may be produced within the digestive tract following bacterial fermentation of food. The former is more commonly associated with brachycephalic dogs, those which gulp their food and those with pharyngeal, oesophageal or respiratory problems. If there is a deficiency in digestive enzymes or ability to absorb nutrients then bacterial fermentation of nutrients may occur leading to flatulence. Some foods are commonly associated with flatulence, including soya bean, legumes, potato, wheat, brassicas, milk and red meat if fed in large amounts. Oral vitamin supplementation may promote bacterial populations and lead to flatulence (Lewis et al., 1987).

Treatment involves identifying and correcting any underlying malabsorption, pharyngeal, oesophageal or respiratory problem. In some cases feeding the animal in a calm environment and two or three times daily will reduce aerophagia. Avoidance of foods known to cause flatulence should also be considered together with feeding a highly-digestible, low-fibre (<2% DM), low-fat (<6% DM) diet (see Table 4.1).

**Table 4.2** Factors which have been implicated in the aetiology of acute pancreatitis in dogs

High-fat diet
Abdominal trauma/surgery
Hypercalcaemia
Drugs; corticosteroids, thiazides, azathioprine
Hyperlipidaemia
Viral infection
Thoracolumbar surgery
Immune mediated disease
Hereditary factors

# Pancreas

## Acute pancreatitis

Acute pancreatitis is more commonly observed in dogs than cats. The aetiology is not fully understood but a large number of predisposing factors have been identified (Table 4.2).

The pancreas has a number of protective mechanisms designed to stop enzyme activation within the gland. The first of these mechanisms is the production of only inactive enzymes within the acinar cells. These enzymes can only be activated by another enzyme called enterokinase found on the brush border of the duodenum. This creates the second protective mechanism, namely that of physical distance between inactive pancreatic enzymes and enterokinase. It is therefore technically impossible for trypsin activation to occur in the acinar cells. The third protective mechanism is the retention of inactive enzymes within zymogen granules, so isolating them from other enzymes in the acinar cells, such as lysosomal enzymes. Lastly, the pancreas produces its own protease inhibitor (pancreatic secretory trypsin inhibitor) which rapidly inactivates any active proteases found in the acinar tissue. This is supported by the presence of protease inhibitors in the plasma, including $\alpha_1$-protease inhibitor and $\alpha_2$-macroglobulin.

How protease enzymes become active in the pancreas remains unclear, but it is thought that zymogen enzymes and lysosomal enzymes may manage to mix and thus activate trypsin. Once activated trypsin is then able to activate itself and many other enzymes produced in the acinar cells.

Phospholipase A hydrolyses lecithin to lysolecithin which causes oedema and necrosis resulting in further release of enzymes. Both phospholipase A and elastase cause major vascular damage in the pancreas, while lipase is responsible for fat necrosis. Amylase is thought to have little involvement in acute pancreatitis. Although the protease inhibitors rapidly bind with trypsin they can be overwhelmed and once this occurs proteases are able to cause systemic damage. Hepatic necrosis, renal tubular damage and inflammation of the stomach, duodenum and transverse colon can occur.

Myocardial depressant factor and enzymes damage the myocardium and promote thrombus formation in the myocardial vessels. Pulmonary oedema follows phospholipase A action on lung membranes (Hall & Macy, 1988).

Clinically animals are presented in a depressed, anorexic state with vomiting, often diarrhoea and acute anterior abdominal pain. Dehydration, shock and collapse will rapidly develop, together with varying degrees of respiratory distress due to pulmonary oedema. Cardiac arrhythmias, jaundice and disseminated intravascular coagulation (DIC) may also develop. Diagnosis is based on clinical signs, radiographic changes and serum chemistry.

Therapy depends on the degree of enzyme activation and tissue damage which has occurred. The majority of cases require IV fluid therapy to correct water and electrolyte losses, such as Ringer's solution. In addition, it is not uncommon for plasma protease inhibitors such as $\alpha_2$-macroglobulin to become depleted. In these cases whole blood or plasma infusions will restore protease inhibitors, help prevent DIC and maintain circulating plasma volume. Pethidine or buprenorphine are valuable as analgesics. Corticosteroids should only be used where shock is thought to be reaching an irreversible stage and the drug is considered to be life saving. Otherwise corticosteroids are contraindicated. Where hyperglycaemia and glycosuria develop, insulin therapy may be required. Antibiotic administration is important when there is extensive peritonitis, to protect against secondary infection.

It is essential that nothing is given *per os*, including water, for at least 3–5 days. Any fluids, food or secretions reaching the stomach and intestine may stimulate pancreatic secretion. In some cases nasogastric aspiration of secretions may further help reduce stimulation of the pancreas. Cimetidine may also effectively reduce gastric secretions.

Once the patient stops vomiting, and at least 3 days have elapsed since initiation of the condition, oral fluids may be provided. If this is tolerated without relapse then a high carbohydrate food may be offered such as pasta, rice or potato. A high carbohydrate diet is recommended at this stage because it has the least stimulating effect on the pancreas (Hall & Macy, 1988). This should be offered as two to three meals/day. If this is tolerated then a highly-digestible low-residue, low-fat (<6% DM) diet may be offered (Table 4.3). This may be supplemented with pancreatic enzyme replacer which helps to reduce the need for full pancreatic function and appears to reduce the pain associated with eating.

Pancreatitis is an unpredictable condition, where a single episode may occur, or repeated bouts referred to as chronic pancreatitis. Where relapsing or chronic pancreatitis occurs, prophylactic treatment using a low-fat diet with added pancreatic enzyme replacer can often be beneficial. However the prognosis must always be guarded, as continual damage can lead to EPI (<15% of cases) in the long term (Hall & Macy, 1988).

### Exocrine pancreatic insufficiency

EPI is more commonly observed in dogs as a congenital disorder within the first 3 years of life, but is rare in cats. A hereditary predisposition exists in the German shepherd dog (Westermark, 1980). It may also occur in older dogs as an acquired condition following repeated episodes of acute pancreatitis with loss of more than 85% of exocrine tissue. In all cases the dogs are literally 'starving in the presence of plenty' because they are unable to make use of the food which has been ingested through a lack of pancreatic digestive enzymes. In up to 70% of cases a secondary bacterial overgrowth develops due to the presence of undigested food in the intestine.

Treatment is expensive and is required for life. Success not only depends on the correct therapeutic regime but substantial owner compliance. Treatment is carried out in three stages. The first stage involves feeding a highly-digestible low-fat (<6% DM) diet at a maintenance level based on the dog's present body weight, together with a suitable enzyme replacer (Table 4.3). This diet should be offered in two meals daily.

Usually within 2 or 3 days the diarrhoea will cease and formed stools will be passed. It is absolutely essential that the dog is fed only the veterinary diet and no other source of food, otherwise the diarrhoea will recur. When formed stools are passed (which will normally occur within 48 hours of initiating the diet), the second stage of treatment may be started. This involves slowly increasing the amount of food and enzyme replacer offered until the dog begins to gain weight while continuing to pass normal faeces (maintenance plus growth). It is rarely necessary to treat the associated bacterial overgrowth as the above regime removes the underlying cause. Usually weight is gained slowly but steadily and it is important not to expect rapid weight gains or diarrhoea will recur (Simpson, 1988).

**Table 4.3** A summary of dietary management which may be of value in patients with pancreatic and hepatic disorders

| Condition | Dietary management |
| --- | --- |
| Acute pancreatitis | Nil by mouth for 4 days; then highly digestible low-fat (<6% DM) diet with added enzyme replacer to aid digestion |
| EPI | Highly-digestible low-fat (<6% DM), low-fibre (<2% DM) diet; feed with adequate levels of enzyme replacer; strict dietary control; feed for maintenance at present body weight to correct diarrhoea, then feed for weight gain; reduce diet and enzyme replacer once the required body weight is achieved |
| Liver disease | Highly-digestible, high-BV protein but in a restricted amount (13–16% DM dogs, and 24–26% DM for cats); increased B vitamins; high energy (as carbohydrate) to meet energy needs and spare protein; may need further protein restriction if the ammonia levels remain high |

Once the dog has attained its optimum body weight, the third stage of treatment involves reducing the amount of diet and enzyme replacer to provide a maintenance level only. In some cases the author has experience of dogs which can maintain their body weight and pass normal faeces on a low-fat veterinary diet and a reduction of up to 70% of enzyme replacer, which significantly reduces the long-term costs. This latter situation can only be attained if a very strict dietary regime is imposed with no variations in the diet type, amount and time of feeding. At present it is unclear how such dogs maintain their body weight on such small amounts of enzyme replacer.

## Liver disease

The liver has a large functional reserve and signs of liver failure only occur when more than 70% of the liver is damaged. Marked regeneration is also possible so long as the basic framework is left intact and there is an adequate blood supply. For these reasons detection of liver disease can present a major diagnostic challenge to the clinician. Many of the clinical signs associated with liver disease are not pathognomonic and may be observed in other conditions. Icterus, hepatomegaly, anterior abdominal pain, ascites and ptyalism in cats are more specific signs associated with liver disease.

The liver plays an important role in the metabolism of protein, fats, carbohydrates, vitamins and minerals. Amino acids, monosaccharides, medium chain triglyceride (MCT) and water-soluble vitamins are absorbed into the portal vein and travel to the liver. The long chain triglyceride (LCT) and fat-soluble vitamins are absorbed into the lacteals and travel via the lymphatic system to the general circulation and eventually to the liver.

Glycogen production and storage normally provides an immediate source of glucose to maintain blood levels. This function is often lost in portosystemic shunts and advanced liver disease, such as cirrhosis, and is more likely to be lost in any hepatic condition where anorexia is also present. In an attempt to meet circulating glucose requirements in liver failure after glycogen stores have been exhausted, gluconeogenesis is employed. In many situations this mechanism fails and hypoglycaemia still occurs. Tissue protein is broken down to supply energy, consequently there is a marked increase in the levels of nitrogen waste requiring conversion to urea and excretion via the kidneys. To this load must be added the ammonia absorbed from the intestine and reaching the liver via the portal blood. In many advanced forms of liver disease such as cirrhosis and in portosystemic shunts, the urea cycle fails and ammonia builds up in the circulation and crosses the blood–brain barrier (BBB) where it can cause marked central nervous signs.

In hepatic disease the plasma amino acid concentration increase, and in particular the level of aromatic amino acids (tryptophan, tyrosine and phenylalanine) compared with the branch-chained amino acids (BCAA: leucine, isoleucine and valine). The breakdown of body protein releases large amounts of amino acids into the circulation but in liver failure metabolism of aromatic amino acids fails so the plasma concentration of these increases (Laflamme, 1988; Bauer, 1986). This is compounded in porto-systemic shunts where absorbed amino acids bypass the liver and further increase plasma levels. BCAA are an important source of energy and protein for skeletal and cardiac muscle and for the brain (Laflamme, 1988). The high levels of aromatic amino acids readily cross the BBB and result in high levels of aromatic amines at nerve terminals which act as false neuro-transmitters competing with natural transmitters. Dietary methionine is converted in the intestine by bacteria to mercaptans which, following absorption, are normally efficiently removed from the portal vein by the liver. Where liver function is impaired high circulating levels of mercaptans exist and act synergistically with ammonia to produce central nervous signs.

The cat is unable to synthesize arginine so dietary requirements are high in order to service the urea cycle. In liver disease this demand is further increased because of tissue catabolism. If the cat is also anorexic, hyper-ammonaemia rapidly develops with accompanying central nervous signs (Center, 1986). In addition to being unable to metabolize amino acids, in advanced liver disease there is also failure to synthesize various important proteins including albumin, prothrombin, $\alpha_1$-anti-trypsin, ceruloplasmin and transferrin (Bauer, 1986).

Fatty acids in the liver are formed into triglyceride, attached to apo-protein B, phospholipid and cholesterol, resulting in the formation of very low density lipoprotein (VLDL). It is thought that lipoprotein deficiency or an inadequate release mechanism of VLDL causes the accumulation of fat in the liver. High levels of fat may further compromise liver function by interfering with ammonia conversion to urea. In addition in many cases of liver disease cholestasis or reduced bile flow means fat digestion and absorp-tion are impaired, resulting in steatorrhoea and diarrhoea. It also means there will be decreased absorption of fat-soluble vitamins.

The aims of therapy in liver disease are to:

1   Find and if possible remove the underlying cause.
2   Prevent further anorexia which compounds the effects of liver failure.
3   Reduce the need for the liver to carry out gluconeogensis, deamination, lipid oxidation and bile secretion.
4   Reduce the levels of circulating ammonia, aromatic amino acids and mercaptans.

Initially an IV infusion of dextrose saline may help correct any dehydra-tion. If the appetite cannot be stimulated then enteral feeding should be considered (see Chapter 5), but no matter which route is chosen the diet must be carefully selected.

A low-protein diet should be offered providing approximately 2 g/kg/day for dogs and 3.5 g/kg/day for cats (see Table 4.3). The protein should be of high biological value (BV), highly digestible and fed in small frequent meals, thus ensuring all the protein is digested and absorbed in the small intestine so that little reaches the colon where ammonia can be produced (Strombeck & Guilford, 1990d). If this level of protein does not reduce the signs of encephalopathy a further reduction to 1.5 g/kg/day may be considered in the dog. However this may have a negative effect as regeneration of hepatic tissue requires an adequate level of dietary protein which may not be satisfied at this low level. Drug therapy can be used to assist in controlling circulating ammonia levels. Oral neomycin and lactulose will effectively reduce ammonia levels while allowing adequate protein to be fed. Where ascites due to hypoproteinaemia is present then a higher level of protein may be required in the diet (>2 g/kg/day). Cottage cheese, egg and milk casein are good protein sources in hepatic disease. These proteins are also high in BCAA and lower in aromatic amino acids thus helping to correct the plasma amino acid profile (Magne & Chiapella, 1986). This is important as aromatic amino acids can only be broken down by the liver and so should be fed in reduced amounts when treating liver failure.

Energy in both dogs and cats should be provided by carbohydrate rather than fat. The carbohydrate must be highly digestible ensuring none reaches the colon where bacterial fermentation can occur. Boiled rice provides the ideal source of carbohydrate in liver disease (Strombeck & Guildford 1990d; Center, 1986).

B vitamins are used as coenzymes by the liver and should be given in increased amounts in liver disease to ensure they do not further compromise liver function.

## Renal failure

The dog and cat are both provided with a large functional reserve of renal tissue. Unfortunately the kidneys have poor powers of regeneration and once nephrons have been destroyed they are not replaced. Renal failure only occurs once 70% or more of the nephrons have been destroyed. At this time signs of polydipsia, polyuria, and the varying signs of vomiting, anorexia, diarrhoea, weight loss and hypoalbuminaemia may develop. If there are adequate numbers of surviving nephrons, they may hypertrophy allowing a return to normal renal function. In such cases the animal is said to have compensated renal disease. There is a limit to such compensation and eventually glomerular filtration and tubular function become inadequate leading to azotaemia and terminal renal disease (Markwell, 1988).

In renal failure the normal products of protein metabolism are not effectively removed by the kidneys and accumulate in the circulation. The azotaemia which develops has a profound effect on other body systems, particularly the gastro-intestinal tract and central nervous system (CNS), leading to vomiting, diarrhoea and occasionally convulsions. In addition there is an increased loss of amino acids in the urine which further increases the demand for protein. Water-soluble vitamins and calcium are also lost from the kidneys but phosphorus is usually retained. The circulating calcium:phosphorus ratio may alter considerably from 1.5:1 to 1:4. Transient hypocalcaemia in association with hyperphosphataemia stimulates parathyroid hormone release, referred to as secondary renal hyper-parathyroidism. The raised parathormone level attempts to correct the hypocalcaemia by resorption of calcium from the bones. Ultimately this resorption can lead to renal osteodystrophy which particularly affects the mandible causing 'rubber jaw'. In addition it is thought that parathormone may contribute to the neurotoxicity oberved in renal failure. Many cases of renal failure develop hypernatraemia and the retention of sodium may be associated with the development of hypertension in these cases.

## Chronic renal failure

In chronic renal failure (CRF) the aim of therapy is to provide a low-protein diet, replace the water-soluble vitamins and calcium which have been lost and prevent accumulation of phosphorus and sodium (Polzin & Osborne, 1987).

A low-protein diet helps to reduce both the accumulation of nitrogenous waste, and the intake of phosphorus which is high in meat. It has also been suggested that restriction of dietary protein and/or phosphorus may affect the rate of progression of renal disease, although this remains a controversial area. The ideal level of protein has not been established in clinical studies; however it has been recommended that dogs with mild to moderate CRF be fed approximately 2.0–2.2 g of high quality protein/kg body weight/day. This should be considered a starting point, and adjustments made to suit the individual case to try to ameliorate clinical and biochemical manifestations of uraemia, whilst avoiding protein malnutrition (Polzin & Osborne, 1986). Protein requirements of cats with renal failure are not known, however, an intake of approximately 3.3–3.5 g protein/kg body weight/day has been recommended for this species (Osborne & Polzin, 1983) (Table 4.4). A number of veterinary diets with restricted protein and phosphorus content designed to assist in the medical management of CRF in dogs and cats are available to the clinician.

Although these diets significantly reduce the phosphorus intake by renal

**Table 4.4** A summary of dietary requirements which may be of value in dogs and cats with renal disease

| | |
|---|---|
| Chronic renal failure | Low protein (2–2.2 g/kg dogs and 3.3–3.5 g/kg cats) of high BV; reduced phosphorus; increased B vitamins; ensure adequate fat and carbohydrate to meet energy requirements and spare protein |
| Glomerular nephritis | Low protein (2 g/kg dogs and 3.5 g/kg cats); of high BV; reduced sodium (<0.3% DM) |
| Acute renal failure | Oliguria phase use low-protein diet at 1.5 g/kg for dogs, use IV dextrose solutions (25%) to provide energy; polyuric phase treat as for CRF above |

patients, this can be further enhanced by giving aluminium hydroxide orally to chelate the phosphorus in the diet thus reducing absorption from the intestine. Use aluminium hydroxide with caution especially in the cat, starting within the range 30–90 mg/kg/day (Polzin & Osborne, 1986). Calcium supplements should only be provided once the calcium : phosphorus ratio has been restored. If calcium supplements are provided too early, soft tissue calcification may develop.

Fat and carbohydrate should be used to provide all the calorie requirements of dogs and cats. This will help to reduce tissue catabolism, weight loss and nitrogen waste accumulation. Fat in particular is valuable because of its calorie density and ability to improve the palatability of low-protein diets. This is most important in the anorexic patient.

**Glomerular nephritis**

In glomerular nephritis hypoalbuminaemia develops because of the persistent proteinuria which exists. When albumin levels fall to less than 15 g/l ascites, hydrothorax and subcutaneous oedema may develop. The presence of these signs also depends on the degree of hypertension present. Due to the hypertension and reduced osmotic pressure, fluid leaves the circulation, reducing blood volume, and stimulates the renin–angiotensin–aldosterone mechanism. This in turn increases retention of sodium and water. Nephrotic syndrome occurs as an end stage of these changes, where proteinuria is severe and accompanied by marked weight loss and fluid retention.

The object of therapy in these cases, in addition to drugs, should be to prevent further accumulation of sodium and water, reduce hypertension, increase serum albumin levels and maintain blood urea levels within the normal range.

A veterinary diet containing no more than 0.3% DM sodium will help reduce fluid retention and reduce hypertension. The diet should also provide approximately 2 g/kg/day for dogs and 3.5 g/kg/day for cats of protein (Polzin & Osborne, 1986) (see Table 4.4). However, protein intake should be maintained at as high a level as the patient will tolerate in order to help restore plasma albumin levels. A high BV protein source such as egg can be added to the veterinary diet, so long as blood urea and proteinuria are carefully monitored. If the protein content of the diet is too high this will worsen the proteinuria and may elevate the blood urea level. Increased dietary protein increases renal blood flow in both dogs and cats and sustained hyperfiltration resulting from this may damage the glomerular micro-vasculature further (Jergens, 1987). The result may be further increases in glomerular permeability and proteinuria. For this reason low-protein diets may slow the progression of renal disease. However a balance must be made between low protein levels for the above reason and higher protein levels to correct the hypoalbuminaemia.

## Congestive heart failure

The prognosis in congestive heart failure is usually guarded but it does depend on the underlying cause and extent of the individual problem, especially with regard to the underlying cardiac pathology and concurrent organ involvement (liver and kidneys). The aggressiveness of treatment will also affect the prognosis.

In congestive heart failure there is activation of the renin–angiotensin–aldosterone mechanism due to low blood pressure and poor renal perfusion. This results in the retention of sodium and water which presents a further volume overload on the failing heart. Pulmonary congestion and oedema may develop and sometimes ascites and hydrothorax are seen. This development is often compounded by release of anti-diuretic hormone (ADH) which leads to further water retention (Ralston, 1989). Where ascites is present this should not be removed by paracentesis unless pressure on the diaphragm is causing respiratory difficulties. Continual fluid removal by paracentesis depletes valuable protein which will be conserved if diuretics are used instead. Cardiac drugs and diuretics may in the long term lead to depletion of serum potassium levels, which must be monitored to determine if supplementation is required.

Protein calorie malnutrition may occur in heart failure as a consequence of several important factors. Patients are often anorexic and malabsorption may occur due to poor intestinal perfusion with changes to villus architecture. Tissue metabolism may be reduced as a result of hypoxia, and increased intestinal permeability can lead to hypoalbuminaemia and some degree of malabsorption. The basal metabolic rate and tissue respiration may increase. The net result of these factors is often weight loss which may be marked in some patients.

Reduced cardiac output also affects the function of the liver and kidneys which may already be compromised, especially in the elderly patient. In addition to hypokalaemia there is some degree of prerenal uraemia which may result in reduced ability to handle nitrogen waste. This may be exacerbated by excessive tissue catabolism increasing the amount of nitrogen waste which must be eliminated. Hepatic congestion is common in congestive heart failure and may be accompanied by some degree of hepatic dysfunction.

Drugs such as digoxin have no direct effect on nutritional requirements. However, diuretics may have a marked effect on sodium and potassium balance. Both frusemide and thiazide diuretics when used long term may cause potassium depletion. If the patient is also anorexic the speed of this fall may be rapid. Spironolactone tends to conserve potassium, and excretes sodium and water. When this drug is used it is important not to restrict the sodium content of diet or sodium depletion will occur. Captopril and enalapril are often used as vasodilators, they reduce aldosterone levels which in turn cause a loss of sodium and retention of potassium. So again low-salt diets should be used with great care when these drugs are used. Hydralazine is an arteriolar dilator, activating aldosterone and causing retention of sodium and water with a loss of potassium, which again influences the type of diet which can be fed (Ralston, 1989).

The emphasis of therapy in congestive heart failure should be to reduce the load on the heart using a combination of drugs, cage rest and diet. Diet itself does not have a primary role in treatment, although it should complement drug therapy.

Exercise and excitement must be strictly reduced and ideally cage rest should be provided in the initial stages. Diuretics and cardiac drugs will reduce the load on the heart and improve tissue perfusion. The aim of dietary management in heart failure is to maintain the lean body mass, reduce the pulmonary oedema and ascites and maintain adequate levels of protein, vitamins and minerals. Dietary management may also help in preventing major electrolyte disturbances, especially with regard to sodium and potassium. Diet should provide all the essential nutrients and calories in a readily digestible form and correct any deficiency states which exist. If the patient is obese, correction of this problem should be rapidly carried out (see section on obesity).

In general a veterinary diet should be used which is low in sodium, moderate in protein but of high BV, and which contains additional vitamins. However, protein levels of more than 30% DM for cats and 18–21% DM for dogs have also been suggested (Ware, 1992). The sodium content of the diet should contain no more than 0.25% DM, and the potassium content should be 0.8–1.5% DM for both dogs and cats (Ralston, 1989).

Low salt and protein diets are often less palatable and as many patients are anorexic it is important to stimulate appetite by making the diet more palatable. The diet should be changed slowly to reduce palatability problems, especially with cats and older patients. It may help to warm food, flavour enhancers such as garlic or tuna may be used if required. Several small meals should be fed daily. If oral intake is inadequate consideration should be given to enteral feeding techniques.

Foods known to be rich in salt, such as cheese, bread, processed meats, cereals, carrots, heart, liver, kidney, whole egg and pet treats should be avoided. Most commercial pet foods have a sodium content (typical range 0.26–0.8% DM) which is high relative to the minimum requirement for adult maintenance. Foods low in salt include beef, rabbit, chicken, horse meat, egg yolk, oatmeal, rice and pasta.

## Feline lower urinary tract disease

Research in recent years has led to improvement in understanding of both the causes of feline lower urinary tract disease (FLUTD) and the categories of disease in which dietary modification may play a role either in management or subsequent prevention of recurrence.

One prospective study of 143 cats with FLUTD conducted in the USA (Osborne et al., 1989b) was able to establish specific causes of disease in just under half of the cases seen, 54% being classified as idiopathic. Uroliths were present in approximately 21% of cases and urethral plugs in a further 22%. Urinary tract infection accounted for only four cases, two of which also had uroliths. Of all these cases a clear rationale for dietary management can only be made for those associated with uroliths or urethral plugs. It must be understood that this is further limited to specific mineral types, where nutritional research has enabled an understanding to be developed of appropriate dietary measures that need to be adopted. Currently this understanding is limited to conditions associated with the presence of struvite (magnesium ammonium phosphate), although research is progressing with regard to other mineral types.

Surveys have shown that struvite is the most common mineral found in feline uroliths with 64.5% of uroliths containing 70–100% of this mineral. However, approximately a further 20% of uroliths are calcium oxalate, and there is some evidence that this proportion is increasing. Struvite is also the most common mineral component of urethral plugs (81.4%), although another 7.4% of these are predominently matrix (Osborne et al., 1992).

The rationale for dietary management of struvite-associated FLUTD has been developed over many years of research which have focused on three major areas: the mineral content of diets, their effect on water turnover in the cat, and their effect on urinary pH. As a result of this research, regime for both dissolution and subsequent prevention of reformation of struvite uroliths have been developed.

The situation in cats with urethral plugs is different for two reasons. Firstly, in the series presented by Osborne *et al.* (1989b) all urethral plugs were associated with urinary tract obstruction and measures to urgently re-establish urethral patency are required. In these cases relatively long-term dietary measures to try to 'dissolve' obstructing material are clearly inappropriate, and thus any role of dietary modification is limited to measures designed to prevent recurrence of disease. Secondly, it should be remembered that dietary modification is only likely to affect formation of struvite as the mineral component of the urethral plug. The origins of the matrix component of the plug are currently unknown, and there is no evidence to suggest that diet affects it. Whether dietary modification can prevent recurrence of FLUTD caused by urethral plugs is not yet clear, and is likely to be dependent on the presence or absence of struvite in the plug. Some evidence supporting the role of dietary modification in the control of FLUTD associated with urethral plugs comes from a study by Filippich (1993). In this study cats which had mostly shown multiple bouts of disease over the previous 18 months showed no recurrence when fed a veterinary diet over a 48-week period.

The aim of dietary management in struvite-associated FLUTD is to create urine which is undersaturated with regard to the components of struvite. In this state no crystallization will occur and preformed crystals will dissolve (Buffington, 1988). The dietary measures that can be adopted include feeding diets that result in an acid urine pH, enhance urine volume, and reduce magnesium intake (Table 4.5). A key factor in control of struvite crystallization on both theoretical and experimental grounds is urine pH (Buffington, 1988; Taton *et al.*, 1984; Tarttelin, 1987). Thus protocols for the management or prevention of recurrence of disease should focus on this aspect, although the other factors mentioned above should not be ignored.

A positive correlation has been reported between number of struvite crystals and pH, with only small quantities of crystals detected at pH values <6.5 (Rich & Kirk, 1969), thus indicating a possible target for acidification. DL-methionine and ammonium chloride are the most widely studied acidifiers in cats. The recommended doses are: DL-methionine 0.2–1 g orally o.d.; ammonium chloride 20 mg/kg orally b.i.d. (Lage *et al.*, 1988).

Both these acidifiers can be toxic and thus care should be taken with dosage. Ching *et al.* (1989) reported indications of chronic acidosis in

**Table 4.5** A summary of dietary requirements which may be of value in cats and dogs with urolithiasis

| | |
|---|---|
| *FLUTD* | Diet should create an acid urine with increased urine volume and reduced levels of magnesium |
| *Canine urolithiasis*<br>Struvite | Reduced protein, magnesium, phosphate and an increased sodium level in diet; urine should become acid |
| Ammonium urate | Reduced protein (<11% DM) diet which creates an alkaline urine; may require to use 1 g sodium bicarbonate/5 kg body weight t.i.d. to create alkaline urine; allopurinol 10 mg/kg t.i.d. |
| Cystine | Diet as for ammonium urates; penicillamine 15 mg/kg b.i.d. |
| Oxalate | Diet as for ammonium urates with reduced calcium and phosphates; hydrochlorthiazide 2–4 mg/kg b.i.d.; potassium citrate 100–150 mg/kg/day |

cats from ad lib feeding of a diet containing 1.5% ammonium chloride (dry matter) for 6 months. This gave rise to an increase in blood-ionized calcium, perhaps mobilized from bone, and resulted in negative net calcium balance for the first 3 months. There were, however, no overt detrimental physical effects within the study period. Methionine can also be toxic, and feeding 2 g/cat/day for 20 days resulted in anorexia, ataxia, cyanosis, methaemoglobinaemia and Heinz body formation leading to haemolytic anaemia (Maede, 1985).

Acidifiers should be given at the time of feeding to be effective and urinary pH measured approximately 4–6 hours after feeding to check for prevention of the alkaline tide effect (Fig. 4.1). It is likely that if this can

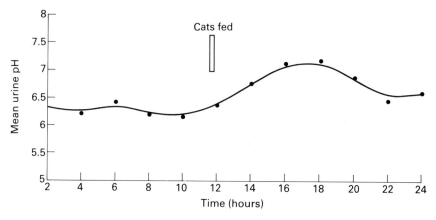

**Fig. 4.1** An example of alkaline tide associated with meal feeding. Measurements taken from four cats. (Data from Waltham Centre for Pet Nutrition studies.)

be prevented by the chosen dose of acidifier, then the urine will remain consistently acid (Polzin & Osborne, 1984). Acidified diets should not be used in cats that have had urinary tract obstruction until any effects of obstruction on acid/base balance in the cat have been corrected.

Whilst evidence indicates that urinary acidification is likely at present to be the cornerstone in the management and subsequent prevention of struvite formation in susceptible cats, other dietary factors should also be addressed.

Measures should be taken to achieve a high urine output, and the easiest method of achieving this is to feed a highly-digestible (to reduce faecal volume and faecal water loss), high-moisture content diet. The benefits of enhancing water turnover were shown in a study in which significant haematuria observed in cats fed a high level of magnesium was almost completely abolished when water intake was increased by feeding the same diet as a slurry containing 80% water (Holme, 1977).

The diet chosen should also provide a relatively low magnesium intake for the cat, and it is important to note that magnesium content should be compared on the basis of ME or DE content, as this actually determines intake.

A number of veterinary diets are available which address some or all of these issues, and these provide a simple, convenient alternative to the adjustment of the cat's normal diet, and to the addition of acidifiers.

The measures described are relevant specifically to struvite and, as noted above, other mineral types may occur in uroliths, and occasionally in urethral plugs. Unfortunately, as noted by Osborne *et al.* (1989b), medical protocols for the dissolution of other types of urolith have not been developed, and of the measures described above, only enhancement of urine volume would be likely to be generally beneficial. Certainly, measures such as acidification and magnesium restriction may be quite inappropriate for the management of some types of non-struvite urolith. It is, therefore, important that efforts are made to identify the type of mineral present in a urethral plug or urolith prior to embarking on a specific management programme. Guidance for 'guesstimating' mineral composition can be found in a number of standard texts.

## Canine urolithiasis

Up to 2% of the canine population may develop urolithiasis. Struvite calculi are formed from magnesium ammonium phosphate crystals in a protein matrix. They are by far the most frequently found calculi in the dog, accounting for 98% of calculi in females and 45% of calculi in males. Other calculi found in the dog include cystine, oxalate and urate in descending order of frequency.

The formation of calculi depends on several factors including:

**1** The presence of mucoproteins which form a non-crystalline matrix for the crystals.

**2** Supersaturation of mineral in the urine usually leading to crystal formation and subsequent calculi development.

**3** Urine pH.

**4** The retention of the crystals in the bladder long enough to allow formation of calculi.

**5** Urease-producing bacteria, especially *Proteus* and *Staphylococcus* spp., which raise the urinary pH and predispose to the formation of struvite calculi. In the case of cystine, oxalate and urate calculi, on the other hand, urinary tract infection (UTI) occurs as a consequence of calculi formation.

**6** Cystine calculi are associated with a hereditary defect in renal function which is most often seen in male dogs. The exact mechanism of cystine urolith formation is not known but dogs with cystinuria have normal plasma cystine levels and normally filter cystine through the glomerulus into the renal tubule. However much smaller amounts of cystine are resorbed by the proximal tubule and in some cases there is also a loss of lysine in the urine.

**7** Ammonium urate calculi are seen most frequently in Dalmatians (60%) due to their inability to excrete allantoin. Urate calculi may also be seen in dogs with portosystemic shunts or liver failure.

In normal dogs urates are formed from degradation of nucleic acids and are then converted into allantoin by the liver. In Dalmatians there is a deficiency in the enzyme hepatic uricase resulting in the excretion of urates in the urine unchanged (Senior, 1989). Urates being relatively insoluble precipitate in urine as uric acid or ammonium urate.

The presence of ammonium biurates in the urine deposit usually indicates an underlying hepatic problem. In particular, biurates are seen in portosystemic shunts or cirrhosis of the liver. So the presence of urate crystals in breeds other than Dalmatians suggests hepatic disease.

The types and characteristics of calculi include those shown in Table 4.6. Struvite crystals/calculi occur most frequently in females. Cystine, oxalate and urate crystals are seen most frequently in males and often obstruct the urethra at the ischial arch or os penis. Oxalate tend to be more common in older dogs.

**Table 4.6** Calculi types and characteristics

| Calculi | Urine acidity | Radiodensity | Texture/shape |
|---------|---------------|--------------|---------------|
| Struvite | Alkaline | Radiodense | Smooth round |
| Cystine | Acid | Radiolucent | Smooth small |
| Oxalate | Acid/alkaline | Radiodense | Rough round/oval |
| Urates | Acid/alkaline | Radiolucent | Smooth shaped |

Treatment of urinary calculi may be achieved by:

1 Surgical removal of the calculi from the bladder and/or urethra.

2 Dietary and drug management aimed at dissolving the calculi and preventing their recurrence. This method is only suitable in cases where there is no immediate risk of urethral obstruction.

The choice depends on the extent of the problem. Those cases presenting with complete urethral obstruction are true emergencies requiring urgent cystocentesis and surgery.

Where medical treatment appears appropriate, it is most important to definitively diagnose the type of calculi present. This ensures the correct type of therapy is instigated. Factors which can assist in this determination include: the radiodensity of the calculi, the pH of the urine, the type of crystal found in the urine deposit and its quantitative analysis, the breed and sex of the dog, and bacteriological examination of urine.

In general the objective of medical therapy is to increase urine production and so reduce urine concentration. This can be acheived by using a moist diet and by adding salt to the diet at 1 g/5 kg body weight t.i.d., or by providing a suitable veterinary diet which contains additional salt (see Table 4.5). Water should always be supplied ad lib, diuretics may also be of value.

**Specific therapy**

*Struvite*

Use one of the veterinary diets which is indicated for this condition and which contains reduced protein, magnesium and phosphate levels. Such a diet contains increased levels of sodium and will also acidify the urine. If such a diet is used it is important not to prescribe additional salt or urinary acidifiers as they are already present in the diet. UTI should be treated following bacteriological culture and sensitivity testing in order to select the most appropriate antibiotic. Dissolution occurs within 2–3 months with this regime. Regular checks should be performed for UTI, urine pH and crystal formation.

*Ammonium urate*

Assuming there is no urinary tract obstruction caused by the small uroliths and no underlying hepatic disease, use a veterinary diet with restricted protein (<11% DM) and minerals, which results in the production of an alkaline urine. If the diet alone does not produce an alkaline urine 1 g sodium bicarbonate/5 kg body weight t.i.d. can be added (Senior, 1989). Specific drug therapy involves preventing uric acid formation using allopurinol 10 mg/kg t.i.d. This drug must be used with caution in uraemic patients as the kidneys are the normal route of excretion (Osborne *et al.*, 1990).

*Cystine*

A similar diet to that used for ammonium urates may also be fed to these patients. If the urine does not become alkaline, sodium bicarbonate can be added as described above. There is some evidence which suggests that sodium may enhance cystinuria and for this reason it may be worth considering the use of potassium citrate to create an alkaline urine instead of sodium bicarbonate (Osborne *et al.*, 1989a). Low-protein diets may reduce the level of cystinuria especially if they contain less cystine and methionine. However the low protein diet is thought to actually reduce the urea concentration of urine which in turn reduces cystinuria. Specific drug therapy using penicillamine at 15 mg/kg b.i.d. binds with cystine and prevents its excretion.

*Oxalate*

Use the same veterinary diet as recommended for control of ammonium urate crystals which not only has a restricted protein content but should also have reduced calcium and phosphate levels. Hydrochlorthiazide at 2–4 mg/kg b.i.d. may reduce calcium excretion and so calcium oxalate formation. Salt must *not* be added to the diet as this reduces the effect of the thiazide diuretic. Potassium citrate at 100–150 mg/kg/day in divided doses will chelate with calcium in an alkaline urine and may reduce intestinal absorption of calcium from the intestine (Bush, 1991). Dietary supplements of vitamin C and D should be avoided as the former is a precursor of oxalic acid and the latter increases calcium excretion in urine (Osborne *et al.*, 1990).

## Diabetes mellitus

This is an endocrine disease associated with disturbed protein, carbohydrate and fat metabolism, resulting in hyperglycaemia and ketoacidosis (Milne, 1987).

Diabetes mellitus is more frequently detected in neutered females from middle age onwards (>8 years). An inherited form is seen in keeshunds under 1 year old. There appears to be a genetic predisposition to diabetes mellitus in the cairn and Scottish terrier, poodle, Samoyed, King Charles spaniel, Rottweiler and dachshund. There are three types of diabetes mellitus (Kaneko *et al.*, 1978).

## Type 1

Insulin-dependent diabetes mellitus which is the commonest form seen in small animals. Obesity is not normally associated with this type of diabetes. There is a deficiency of B cells in the islets of Langerhans and thus of insulin secretion. In some cases external factors such as drugs and viral infections may induce a cell-mediated immune response which destroys B cells. Type 1 diabetes may also occur following repeated episodes of acute or chronic pancreatitis. Excess adrenaline produced from rare phaeochromocytomas of the adrenal medulla may also be a cause. Insulin levels are usually low in these cases and glycosuria and ketonuria are usually present.

## Type 2

This form of diabetes mellitus is associated with obesity which results in insulin resistance, hyperinsulinism and reduction in the number of insulin receptor sites. The response to elevated blood sugar and rising insulin levels is poor. As obesity develops, so the level of insulin resistance increases. Eventually other complications develop, such as interference with the transport and metabolism of glucose which culminates in type 2 diabetes mellitus. Excess growth hormone observed in acromegaly or excessive progesterone observed in the oestrus cycle can also result in this type of diabetes. A similar situation occurs when progestogens are administered to control oestrus. Cushing's disease and therapeutic administration of corticosteroids also induce type 2 diabetes mellitus.

As a consequence of insulin resistance the B cells are stimulated resulting in a further elevation of insulin levels. Where cases are left untreated, B cell exhaustion occurs and type I diabetes mellitus develops. Obesity is often associated with these cases and glycosuria and ketonuria are often detected.

## Type 3

This occurs where the patient has an abnormal glucose tolerance without clinical signs of diabetes mellitus. This may be associated with the early stages of type 1 or type 2 diabetes mellitus. These cases may be associated with obesity.

Therapy in diabetes mellitus depends on the type of disease present and the detection of any underlying cause such as Cushing's disease, acromegaly, hypothyroidism, drug administration such as progestogens and corti-costeroids, and also whether the animal is neutered. Where the animal is obese, a reduction in body weight increases the number of insulin receptor

**Table 4.7** A summary of the dietary requirements which may be of value in diabetes mellitus and hyperlipidaemia in dogs

| | |
|---|---|
| Diabetes mellitus | Protein 25–30% DM of high BV; fat reduced (<10% DM), but increased carbohydrate (45–50% DM) and high fibre (10–15% DM) |
| Hyperlipidaemia | Low-fat (<6% DM), high-fibre (>10% DM) diet |

sites and reduces the diabetic effect. In type 3 diabetes, dietary management and oral hypoglycaemic drugs may be used. However, the majority of diabetic patients require insulin therapy in association with strict dietary management.

Home-made diets should be avoided because they are rarely consistent, and a veterinary diet should be used. Where the animal is obese then control of diabetes mellitus and weight loss can be achieved using a reducing diet. Where the animal has lost weight a higher calorie diet should be used. The important feature is absolute consistency in composition, amounts fed and timing of feeding.

The diet should be low in fat (<10% DM) and contain a moderate amount of protein (ideally 25–30% DM) with a high BV. Diets containing high levels of complex carbohydrate (45–50% DM), e.g. maize or rice starch are now recommended (Wolter, 1989). In addition, dietary fibre (approximately 10–13% DM) is indicated to decrease the rate of absorption from the small intestinal lumen (Table 4.7). Soluble fibres (e.g. guar) have been found to have a potent effect in slowing intestinal absorption of glucose, and some evidence also suggests a relationship with increased sensitivity to insulin (Milne, 1987). Only low levels of soluble fibre are recommended. Such a regime aims to reduce postfeeding surges in blood sugar levels which the diabetic patient finds difficult to tolerate.

Snacks or *any* changes in the type, quality and quantity of diet should not be permitted, especially during the stabilization period.

Exercise should be encouraged, but extreme variations from day to day should be avoided as they will affect the blood sugar and insulin requirements.

The daily routine should involve:

1   Collection of an early morning urine sample.

2   Measurement of glucose and ketones in the urine. Where readily available, blood sugar can be measured instead and is more accurate.

3   Calculation of the daily insulin requirement.

(a)  Initially 0.5 IU/kg of 24 hour insulin should be given subcutaneously.

(b)  Thereafter the daily dose should be adjusted based on urine glucose. If urine glucose is >2% then previous day's dose +2 IU. If urine glucose is 0% then previous day's dose −2 IU. If urine glucose is 0.25% then previous day's dose.

**4**  25% of the daily ration should be fed in the morning.

**5**  Insulin should only be injected if the patient eats this meal.

**6**  The remaining ration should be fed 8 hours later.

Stabilization usually takes approximately 2 weeks and is best carried out in the hospital. Careful records should be kept of all food provided, insulin administered and urine analysed. The daily routine should be strictly adhered to.

Hypoglycaemia may occur when the patient receives too much insulin, fails to eat following injections of insulin, or exercises too strenuously. Signs include weakness, lethargy, ataxia, muscle tremors and eventually convulsions. Where these signs occur and the patient is conscious, chocolate, sugar, honey or standard pet food should be fed to restore blood sugar levels. When convulsions occur it is unwise to offer food and hypoglycaemia should be corrected by IV administration of dextrose solutions. Usually 2–15 ml of 50% dextrose will correct the situation (Nelson, 1992).

## Hyperlipidaemia

Hyperlipidaemic patients are those with fasting lipaemia. Normal animals may be lipaemic following a meal, but fasting lipaemia is abnormal. Hyperlipidaemic plasma appears milky on visual examination. It is associated with both hypercholesterolaemia and hypertriglyceridaemia, and in some cases there may also be abnormalities in plasma lipoproteins (Debowes, 1987).

Hyperlipidaemia may be seen in several endocrine disorders including hypothyroidism, diabetes mellitus and Cushing's disease. It is also seen in acute pancreatitis, chronic renal failure and as an inherited disorder in both dogs and cats (Armstrong & Ford, 1989).

Where possible the underlying cause should be identified and corrected as this will usually resolve the hyperlipidaemia. In idiopathic cases or in inherited cases, dietary management may be of some value in controlling circulating lipid levels. Home-made diets should be avoided as the lipid content will fluctuate from day to day and because suitable veterinary diets are available.

A low-fat (<6% DM), high-fibre (>10% DM) diet may be beneficial in reducing the lipaemia in inherited or idiopathic cases (see Table 4.7). The effect is not only produced by the low fat component but by the fibre, which reduces the assimilation of fat from the intestine and improves insulin receptor activity (Armstrong & Ford, 1989). Veterinary diets are available to meet these requirements for both dogs and cats. Care is needed to ensure the calorie content is not too low, resulting in weight loss when used in the long term. The amounts fed have to be adjusted to take into account the level of lipaemia and body weight of the patient. Recent work has suggested that feeding fish oils may reduce lipid levels (Armstrong & Ford, 1989).

In general a high-fibre diet with <6% fat DM should be chosen. Fibre not only reduces the calorie density but also reduces the absorption of carbohydrate and fat from the intestine. A reduced calorie intake is important to ensure that there is not an excess energy input as this would be converted to lipid which would be retained in the circulation, exacerbating the problem.

## Eclampsia

Eclampsia occurs most frequently in bitches with large litters of puppies between 3 and 6 weeks old. The condition is more common in the small breeds although any breed may be affected. The clinical signs are associated with lowering of serum calcium levels and include muscle tremors, ataxia and, in severe cases, convulsions.

Treatment depends on the severity in individual cases. Where clinical signs are severe, IV calcium borogluconate should be given. Where clinical signs are less acute, oral calcium supplements may be used.

In addition to the treatment described above, it is important to examine the overall management of the lactating bitch. Puppies from 3 weeks of age should be encouraged to take solid food and so reduce the demand for milk from the bitch. In addition the lactating bitch has a very large demand for energy and other nutrients. This cannot be satisfied with low-calorie density diets as it will be physically impossible for the bitch to consume enough of the diet to meet all her nutritional requirements. For this reason a high calorie density diet designed for lactating animals should be fed. This diet should be fed ad lib so the bitch does not have to consume very large amounts of food at set times each day.

As an example a Labrador bitch with a large litter of puppies will require approximately 1500 kcal (6.3 MJ) ME for maintenance and a further 5000–5500 kcal (20 920–23 MJ) for milk production at the peak of lactation. This means that approximately 7000 kcal (29 MJ) of energy must be consumed daily to meet her needs or she will use body reserves to meet nutritional requirements.

## Obesity

Obesity is a condition where a positive energy balance has resulted in excessive accumulation of adipose tissue. Obesity is said to occur when an individual's weight exceeds its optimal weight for breed, sex and age by 15%. The prevalence of obesity lies between 15 and 40% in dogs (Hand *et al.*, 1989) and is thought to be approximately 9% in cats (Anderson, 1973). Obesity is seen more frequently in females and neutered animals; it is more common in geriatric pets as there is a tendency for lean muscle mass to fall and adipose tissue to accumulate with age. Other factors which may be important include obesity in the owner, feeding home-made diets, begging, imbalanced diets, ad lib feeding and offering treats or supplements.

Assessing the degree of obesity can be difficult and various methods have been adopted in the past. Comparison of the pet's present weight with its weight when 1 year old may be helpful. Comparison of present body weight with the accepted weight for the breed, age and sex of the pet concerned is another method. The problem with these methods is that they take no account of physical development which may result in a working dog having a larger muscle mass and thus heavier body weight.

Assessment of body fat on physical examination has also been used to detect obesity. The loss of 'hour glass appearance' when viewed from above, together with increased fat deposits at the tail head in dogs and inguinal region in cats are useful parameters. In addition, the inability to see and feel the ribs may also indicate the presence of obesity (Edney & Smith, 1986).

It is extremely important to examine an obese animal thoroughly to ensure there is no underlying disease process causing increase in body weight (Table 4.8).

Obesity may predispose the dog and cat to a variety of different physical conditions, which would be less likely if they were of normal body weight.

There is an association between obesity and hypertension although the mechanism by which this occurs is not clearly understood. Obesity in itself is unlikely to cause congestive heart failure but the likelihood is increased in those already predisposed to heart disease. Increased pulmonary resistance with reduced respiratory reserve, increased chance of tracheal collapse, increased tissue oxygen demands and hypoventilation may occur.

Surgery is more difficult with tissues coated in fat making dissection and identification difficult. It also appears that postsurgical infection is more likely in obese patients (Crane, 1991).

Secondary hormonal imbalances may also occur in obese pets. Insulin resistance, hyperglycaemia, poor glucose tolerance and impaired release of growth hormone have been recorded (Nelson, 1989).

**Table 4.8** Examine obese patients thoroughly to ensure there is no underlying disease process which has induced apparent weight gain

Abdominal enlargement
  ascites
  pregnancy
  neoplasia
  faeces
Diabetes mellitus
Hyperadrenocorticalism
Acromegaly
Hypothyroidism

Up to 24% of obese pets have concurrent locomotor problems which may be secondary to the increased body weight. Conditions such as cruciate ligament damage, intervertebral disc problems and arthritis are common in obese pets.

Dystocia, infertility, constipation, flatulence and poor heat tolerance may also be observed in obese dogs and cats.

Obesity occurs where there is an excess intake of energy over expenditure. This results in a positive energy balance and ultimately leads to obesity. However the factors which cause a positive energy balance are complex and involve physiological, genetic and environmental factors. In other words, obesity is *not* simply due to greed or overeating. If this were true, then all individuals would respond to a high energy dense diet in the same way, which is rarely the case. Factors involved may include:

1  Inadequate satiety signals.
2  Social pressure.
3  Dietary factors.
4  Neutering.
5  Body energy expenditure.

Hunger is modified by input from stimuli such as distension of the stomach and intestine, the presence of nutrients in the circulation and liver, and the sight, smell and taste of food. These stimuli have a negative feedback effect on the hypothalamus which controls energy intake. No single factor appears to stop food intake, it seems that several factors are required simultaneously (see Chapter 5).

Social pressures including competition between animals may increase food intake. Feeding snacks and begging are other important external factors. Some owners over indulge their pet with treats which are energy dense.

Neutering doubles the likelihood of obesity occurring in either sex. This may be due partly to a reduced energy expenditure following neutering but it is also believed that the loss of the satiety effect of oestrogen or testosterone is important.

Sixty to seventy per cent of consumed energy is used to maintain body functions (homoeostasis), 10% is lost as heat of utilization (specific dynamic effect), and the remaining 20–30% used for physical activity. If physical activity is greatly increased, so appetite will also increase. Where physical activity is reduced no proportional fall in appetite may occur. So in the latter situation a positive energy balance is easily achieved.

There are two types of body fat, white and brown fat. The majority of fat is white (approximately 95%) and only a small amount is brown (approximately 5%). The white fat makes up the major energy store of the the body. The brown fat is used to maintain body temperature and to produce heat. Most brown fat lies subcutaneously round the thoracic region and is well supplied by sympathetic nerves and capillaries. It does not produce adenosine triphosphate (ATP) but uses energy for heat production after food intake, and to maintain body temperature in the neonate. Heat production increases with increased calorie intake, and heat production falls with reduced calorie intake. In this way energy is conserved when in short supply and lost as heat when in excess. Both white and brown fat increase in size when excess calories are consumed and vice versa.

In man obesity occurs as a consequence of an increased size in fat cells (hypertrophic obesity) but it can also occur as a result of increased numbers of fat cells (hyperplastic obesity). The prognosis is much worse in the latter because measures taken to control obesity reduce the fat cell size but *not* their number. Whether this situation occurs in dogs and cats is not yet fully understood.

It appears that the number of fat cells increases only during a specific stage in life, usually during late foetal development and the growth phase. In maturity it is more common for fat cells to increase in size rather than increase in numbers. So to prevent obesity it is important to prevent overfeeding during the growth period (Crane, 1991).

When weight loss occurs, it is achieved by a reduction in fat cell size, but there is a limit to this reduction in cell size. Further weight loss can only occur as a result of loss of muscle mass. So if there are a large number of fat cells present there is a limit to the amount of weight which can be lost. The greater the number of fat cells present, the harder it is to lose weight. Also, the ability to maintain an optimal weight becomes more constrained when there are numerous fat cells present.

**Therapy**

The aim should always be to prevent obesity from occurring rather than to correct it. This can be achieved by client education from their first visit with a new puppy or kitten and through each annual vaccination appointment. Such a scheme will allow the early identification of an overweight puppy or kitten and may prevent the formation of hyperplastic obesity which will predispose the pet to lifelong problems with weight. Careful discussion regarding dietary management and weight control during the growth phase is therefore very important for the long-term well-being of the pet.

When presented with an overweight dog or cat a thorough clinical examination should be carried out before starting on an obesity programme, to ensure there is no underlying disease state causing the weight gain (see Table 4.8).

Assuming the pet is simply obese, it is *very* important to establish owner compliance right at the start of the weight loss programme. Without the owner's cooperation and commitment to the weight loss programme, success will be impossible.

The animal should be weighed using accurate scales and a target weight determined for that individual. One approach is to try to identify an ideal weight based on the breed, age and sex of the individual. However, this may prove difficult in practice, particularly with cross-bred animals, and may also lead to very severe reductions in food allowance if the animal is extremely obese. An alternative is to target for an initial reduction of approximately 15% from the animal's current weight (Edney, 1974), then reassess the situation when this loss is achieved. Although taking longer to complete, advantages of the latter approach are the likely greater accuracy of ideal weight prediction, and improved motivation of the owner by the achievement of one target within a reasonable time frame.

The maintenance energy requirement for the animal at its target weight should then be determined, and it is recommended that the following equations be used.

*Dog*   $125 \times$ weight (kg)$^{0.75} = d$ kcal/day ($\times 4.184 = d_1$ kJ/day)

*Cat*    $60 \times$ weight (kg) $= c$ kcal/day ($\times 4.184 = c_1$ kJ/day)

A proportion of this energy requirement is then used to calculate the amount of food that should be offered. For the dog, feeding levels of 40–60% of maintenance at the target weight have been recommended, with further reductions considered if necessary after careful assessment at intermediate weighings during the period of weight reduction. Weight losses averaging approximately 14% of starting weight have been achieved in 12 weeks by this method, although considerable variability has also been noted (Edney, 1974; Markwell *et al.*, 1990). Severe calorie restriction is contraindicated in cats because of the risk of hepatic lipidosis, thus the health of cats on a weight reduction programme should always be closely monitored. In this species 60–70% of maintenance at the target weight is recommended. Weight losses averaging 13.7% have been recorded over 18 weeks in cats using a slightly higher feeding level than this (Wills *et al.*, 1993).

The amount of food to be offered will be determined by its energy content, and an example of how this may be calculated is given in the equations below.

Dog's target weight $= 20$ kg

Maintenance allowance at target $= 1182$ kcal (4945 kJ)/day

50% of maintenance allowance $= 591$ kcal (2473 kJ)/day

Amount of food/day [assuming 65 kcal (272 kJ)/100 g] $= 909$ g

The chosen diet may either be a modification of the animal's normal food, or a veterinary diet specially formulated for weight reduction. Use of one of the latter products is likely to bring about improved owner compliance, as they are giving a completely new diet to their pet, rather than trying to accurately adjust a pre-existing diet. In addition, long-term feeding of 'normal' foods at substantially reduced intake could result in nutrient deficiencies, as the nutrient levels are balanced to the energy contents of the foods. Some veterinary diets avoid this risk by containing increased levels of essential nutrients. Whichever diet is chosen, it is important to stress to the owner that it must (apart from water) form the sole source of nutrition for the animal. In the case of cats this may necessitate confining them to the home, to prevent either hunting or supplementation of their diets from other sources.

The owner should be encouraged to return to the practice at regular intervals for reweighing of the animal and for an assessment of progress. These sessions provide an opportunity for further encouragement of the owner and discussion of any problems that may have arisen. A graphical recording of weight changes at this time will help to show the owner progress that is being achieved.

Starvation should not be used as a means of weight reduction, because it creates a state of negative nitrogen balance, loss of lean muscle mass and decreased resting metabolic rate (Crane, 1991). In the cat it also puts the animal at risk of hepatic lipidosis. Another drawback is the lack of owner involvement in the process of calorie restriction and weight reduction (the animal is hospitalized), and thus no retraining of them in a regime of careful dietary management for their pet.

Exercise on its own has little effect in reducing obesity because strenuous exercise only uses small amounts of energy. However, exercise does increase the resting metabolic rate and there is a tendency to increase lean muscle mass to cope with the exercise, with a small loss in adipose tissue. If this is combined with a weight loss programme a better and more rapid end result will be achieved. Great care may be required with regard to exercise in pets which are obese but also have concurrent cardiopulmonary or locomotor problems, although even these pets will benefit from mild (but carefully controlled) exercise.

Once the desired weight loss has been achieved it is important to maintain the optimal body weight. Owners should be carefully counselled with regard to feeding and a maintenance diet calculated for them. Initially re-visits should be timetabled every month and if all is going well these can be extended to once every 3 months.

# References

Anderson, R.S. (1973) Obesity in the dog and cat. In *The Veterinary Annual*, pp. 182–186, Grunsell, C.S.G. & Hill, F.W.G. (eds). John Wright, Bristol.

Anderson, R.S. (1982) Nutrition and bone disease in pet animals. *Pedigree Digest*, **9**, 5–12.

Armstrong, P.J. & Ford, R.B. (1989) Hyperlipidaemia. In *Current Veterinary Therapy X*, pp. 1046–1051, Kirk, R.W. (ed.). W.B. Saunders, Philadelphia.

August, J.R. (1985) Dietary hypersensitivity in dogs; cutaneous manifestations, diagnosis and management. *Compendium of Continuing Education for the Practicing Veterinarian*, 7, 469–477.

Bauer, J.E. (1986) Nutrition and liver function; nutrient metabolism in health and disease. *Compendium of Continuing Education for the Practicing Veterinarian*, 8, 923–931.

Bennett, D. (1976) Nutrition and bone disease in the dog and cat. *Veterinary Record*, 98, 313–320.

Buffington, C.A. (1986) Therapeutic use of vitamins in companion animals. In *Current Veterinary Therapy IX*, pp. 40–43, Kirk, R.W. (ed.). W.B. Saunders, Philadelphia.

Buffington, C.A. (1988) Feline struvite urolithiasis: effect of diet. In *Proceedings of the ESVNU Annual Symposium, Barcelona*, pp. 60–112, Intercongress.

Burns, M.G. (1982) Intestinal lymphangectasia in the dog: a case report and review. *Journal of the American Animal Hospital Association*, 18, 97–105.

Burrows, C.F. (1986) Constipation. In *Current Veterinary Therapy IX*, pp. 904–908, Kirk, R.W. (ed.). W.B. Saunders, Philadelphia.

Burrows, C.F. (1988) Diseases of the canine and feline colon and anorectum. In *Proceedings of a Course in Small Animal Gastroenterology and Nutrition*, pp. 225–258, New Zealand Veterinary Association, Auckland.

Burrows, C.F., Bright, R.M. & Spencer, C.P. (1985) Influence of dietary composition on gastric emptying and motility in dogs; potential involvement in acute gastric dilatation. *American Journal of Veterinary Research*, 46, 2609–2612.

Bush, B.M. (1991) The urinary system. In *Canine Medicine and Therapeutics*, pp. 601–658, Chandler, E.A., Thompson, D.J., Sutton J.B. & Price, C.J. (eds). Blackwell Scientific Publications, Oxford.

Carlotti, D.N., Perry, I. & Prost, C. (1990) Food allergy in dogs and cats; a review and report of 43 cases. *Veterinary Dermatology*, 1, 55–62.

Caywood, D., Teague, H.D., Jackson, D.A., Levitt, M.D. & Bond, J.H. (1977) Gastric gas analysis in canine gastric distension-volvulus. *Journal of the American Animal Hospital Association*, 13, 459–462.

Center, S. (1986) Feline liver disorders and their management. *Compendium of Continuing Education for the Practicing Veterinarian*, 8, 889–901.

Ching, S.V., Fettman, M.J., Hamar, D.W., Nayode, L.A. & Smith, K.R. (1989) The effect of chronic acidification using ammonium chloride on acid–base and mineral metabolism in the adult cat. *Journal of Nutrition*, 119, 902–915.

Crane, S.W. (1991) Occurrence and management of obesity in companion animals. *Journal of Small Animal Practice*, 32, 275–282.

Dakin, K.A. (1988) Food allergy in a cat. *Companion Animal Practice*, 2, 10–11.

Debowes, L.J. (1987) Lipid metabolism and hyperlipoproteinaemia in dogs. *Compendium of Continuing Education for the Practicing Veterinarian*, 9, 727–734.

Edney, A.T.B. (1974) Management of obesity in the dog. *Veterinary Medicine Small Animal Clinician* 49, 46–49.

Edney, A.T.B. & Smith, P.M. (1986) Studies of obesity in dogs visiting veterinary practices in the United Kingdom. *Veterinary Record*, 118, 391–396.

Edwards, D.F. & Russell, R.G. (1987) Probable vitamin K deficient bleeding in two cats, with malabsorption syndrome secondary to lymphocytic-plasmacytic enteritis. *Journal of Veterinary Internal Medicine*, 1, 97–101.

Filippich, L.J. (1993) The use of a therapeutic diet in feline lower urinary tract disease (in press).

Hall, E.J. & Batt, R.M. (1988) Challenge studies to demonstrate gluten sensitivity of a naturally occurring enteropathy in Irish setter dogs. *Gastroenterology*, 94, A167.

Hall, J.A., Burrows, C.F. & Twedt, D.C. (1988) Gastric motility in dogs. Part 1: Normal gastric function. *Compendium of Continuing Education for the Practicing Veterinarian*, 10, 1282–1293.

Hall, J.A. & Macy, D.W. (1988) Acute canine pancreatitis. *Compendium of Continuing Education for the Practicing Veterinarian*, 10, 403–416.

Hand, M.S., Armstrong, P.J. & Allen, T.A. (1989) Obesity – occurrence, treatment and prevention. *Veterinary Clinics of North America: Small Animal Practice*, **19**, 447–474.

Hayes, K.C. (1982) Nutritional problems in cats: taurine deficiency and vitamin A excess. *Canadian Veterinary Journal*, **23**, 2–5.

Hinder, R.A. & Kelly, K.A. (1977) Canine gastric emptying of solids and liquids. *American Journal of Physiology*, **233**, E335.

Holme, D.W. (1977) Research into feline urological syndrome. In *The Kal Kan Symposium for the Treatment of Dog and Cat Diseases*, pp. 40–45, Kal Kan, Vernon, CA.

Hoskins, J.D. (1990) Management of faecal impaction. *Compendium of Continuing Education for the Practicing Veterinarian*, **12**, 1579–1585.

Jergens, A.E. (1987) Glomerulonephritis in dogs and cats. *Compendium of Continuing Education for the Practicing Veterinarian*, **9**, 903–908.

Kaneko, J.J., Mattheeuws, D., Rottiers, R.P. & Vermeulen, A. (1978) Glucose tolerance and insulin response in diabetes mellitus of dogs. *Journal of Small Animal Practice*, **19**, 85–94.

Kealy, J.K. & McAllister, H. (1991) Metabolic bone disease. *Waltham International Focus*, **1**, 21–27.

Kennedy, P.C. & Cello, R.M. (1966) Colitis of boxer dogs. *Gastroenterology*, **51**, 926–929.

Laflamme, D.P. (1988) Dietary management of canine hepatic encephalopathy. *Compendium of Continuing Education for the Practicing Veterinarian*, **10**, 1258–1262.

Lage, A.L., Polzin, D.J. & Zenoble, R.D. (1988) Diseases of the bladder. In *Handbook of Small Animal Practice*, pp. 605–619, Morgan, R.H. (ed.). Churchill Livingstone, New York.

Leib, M.S. & Martin, R.A. (1987) Therapy of gastric dilatation-volvulus in dogs. *Compendium of Continuing Education for the Practicing Veterinarian*, **9**, 1155–1163.

Lewis, L.D., Morris, M.L. & Hand, M.S. (1987) Gastrointestinal, pancreatic and hepatic disease. In *Small Animal Nutrition III*, pp. 1–7 Mark Morris Associates, Kansas.

Magne, M.L. & Chiapella, A.M. (1986) Medical management of canine chronic hepatitis. *Compendium of Continuing Education for the Practicing Veterinarian*, **8**, 915–921.

Maede, Y. (1985) Methionine-induced haemolytic anaemia with methaemoglobinaemia and Heinz body formation in erythrocytes in cats. *Journal of the Japanese Veterinary Medical Association*, **38**, 568–571.

Markwell, P.J. (1988) Clinical small animal nutrition. In *Dog and Cat Nutrition*, 2nd edn, pp. 97–116, Edney, A.T.B. (ed.). Pergamon Press, Oxford.

Markwell, P.J., van Erk, W., Parkin, G.D., Sloth, C.J. & Shantz-Christensen, T. (1990) Obesity in the dog. *Journal of Small Animal Practice*, **31**, 533–537.

Milne, E.M. (1987) Diabetes mellitus; an update. *Journal of Small Animal Practice*, **28**, 727–736.

Murdoch, D.B. (1986) Diarrhoea in the dog and cat 1. Acute diarrhoea. *British Veterinary Journal*, **142**, 307–316.

Nelson, R.W. (1989) Dietary therapy for canine diabetes mellitus. In *Current Veterinary Therapy X*, pp. 1008–1009, Kirk, R.W. (ed.). W.B. Saunders, Philadelphia.

Nelson, R.W. (1992) Endocrine disorders. In *Essentials of Small Animal Internal Medicine*, pp. 561–586, Nelson, R.W. & Couto, C.G. (eds). Mosby, St Louis.

Nelson, R.W., Dimperio, M.E. & Long, G.G. (1984) Lymphocytic-plasmacytic colitis in the cat. *Journal of the American Veterinary Medicial Association*, **184**, 1133–1135.

Osborne, C.A., Hoppe, A. & O'Brien, T.D. (1989a) Medical dissolution and prevention of cystine urolithiasis. In *Current Veterinary Therapy X*. pp. 1189–1192, Kirk, R.W. (ed.). W.B. Saunders, Philadelphia.

Osborne, C.A., Kruger, J.P., Lulich, J.P., Bartages, J.W., Polzin, D.J., Molitor, T., Beauclair, K.D. & Onffroy, J. (1992) Feline matrix crystalline urethral plugs: a unifying hypothesis of causes. *Journal of Small Animal Practice*, **33**, 18–23.

Osborne, C.A., Lulich, J.P., Bantgers, J.W. & Felice, L.J. (1990) Medical dissolution and prevention of canine and feline uroliths; diagnosis and therapeutic caveats. *Veterinary Record*, **127**, 369–373.

Osborne, C.A. & Polzin, D.J. (1983) Conservative medical management of feline chronic polyuric renal failure. In *Current Veterinary Therapy VIII*, pp. 1008–1018, Kirk, R.W. (ed.). W.B. Saunders, Philadelphia.

Osborne, C.A., Polzin, D.J., Kruger, J.P., Lulich, J.P., Johnston, G.R. & O'Brien, T.D. (1989b) Relationship of nutritional factors to the cause, dissolution and prevention of feline uroliths and urethral plugs. *Veterinary Clinics of North America: Small Animal Practice*, **19**, 561–581.

Polzin, D.J. & Osborne, C.A. (1984) Medical prophylaxis of feline urinary tract disorders. *Veterinary Clinics of North America: Small Animal Practice*, **14**, 661–675

Polzin, D.J. & Osborne, C.A. (1986) Update – conservative management of chronic renal failure. In *Current Veterinary Therapy IX*, pp. 1167–1173, Kirk, R.W. (ed.). W.B. Saunders, Philadelphia.

Polzin, D.J. & Osborne, C.A. (1987) Dietary management of canine renal failure. *Contemporary Issues in Small Animal Practice*, **4**, 151–176.

Ralston, S.L. (1989) Dietary considerations in the treatment of heart failure. In *Current Veterinary Therapy X*, pp. 302–307, Kirk, R.W. (ed.). W.B. Saunders, Philadelphia.

Rich, L.J. & Kirk, R.W. (1969) The relationship of struvite crystals to urethral obstruction in cats. *Journal of the American Veterinary Medical Association*, **154**, 153–157.

Senior, D. (1989) Medical management of urate uroliths. In *Current Veterinary Therapy X*, pp. 1178–1182, Kirk, R.W. (ed.). W.B. Saunders, Philadelphia.

Sherding, R.G. (1990) Management of constipation and dyschezia. *Compendium of Continuing Education for the Practicing Veterinarian*, **17**, 677–685.

Simpson, J.W. (1988) Treatment of canine exocrine pancreatic insufficiency. *Veterinary Practice*, **20**, 5.

Simpson, J.W. & Else, R.W. (1991a) Conditions of the stomach. In *Digestive Disease in the Dog and Cat*, pp. 60–87, Simpson, J.W. & Else, R.W. (eds) Blackwell Scientific Publications, Oxford.

Simpson, J.W. & Else, R.W. (1991b) Diseases of the small intestine. In *Digestive Disease in the Dog and Cat*, pp. 101–139, Simpson, J.W. & Else, R.W. (eds) Blackwell Scientific Publications, Oxford.

Simpson, J.W. & Else, R.W. (1991c) Diseases of the large intestine. In *Digestive Disease in the Dog and Cat*, pp. 140–169, Simpson, J.W. & Else, R.W. (eds) Blackwell Scientific Publications, Oxford.

Strombeck, D.R. & Guilford, W.G. (1990a) Gastric dilatation, gastric volvulus. In *Small Animal Gastroenterology*, 2nd edn, pp. 228–243, Stonegate Publishing, California.

Strombeck, D.R. & Guilford, W.G. (1990b) Classification, pathophysiology and symptomatic treatment of diarrhoeal diseases. In *Small Animal Gastroenterology*, 2nd edn, pp. 279–295, Stonegate Publishing, California.

Strombeck, D.R. & Guilford, W.G. (1990c) Nutritional management of gastrointestinal disease. In *Small Animal Gastroenterology*, 2nd edn, pp. 690–709, Stonegate Publishing, California.

Strombeck, D.R. & Guilford, W.G. (1990d) Hepatic vascular disease. In *Small Animal Gastroenterology*, 2nd end. pp. 648–671, Stonegate Publishing, California.

Tarttelin, M.F. (1987) Feline struvite urolithiasis: factors affecting urine pH may be more important than magnesium levels in food. *Veterinary Record*, **121**, 227–230.

Taton, G.F., Hamar, D.W. & Lewis, L.D. (1984) Urinary acidification in the prevention and treatment of feline struvite urolithiasis. *Journal of the American Veterinary Medical Association*, **184**, 437–443.

Twedt, D.C. (1983) Disorders of gastric retention. In *Current Veterinary Therapy VIII*, pp. 761–770, Kirk, R.W. (ed.). W.B. Saunders, Philadelphia.

Van der Gaag, I., Toorenburg, J., Voorhoot, G., Happe, R.P. & Aalps, R.H.G. (1978) Histiocytic ulcerative colitis in a French bulldog. *Journal of Small Animal Practice*, **19**, 283–290.

Van Kruiningen, H.J. & Dobbin, W.O. (1979) Feline histiocytic colitis. *Veterinary Pathology*, **16**, 215–222.

Van Kruiningen, H.J., Gregoire, K. & Meuten, D.J. (1974) Acute gastric dilatation. A review of comparative aspects by species and by study in dogs and monkeys. *Journal of the American Animal Hospital Association*, **10**, 294–324.

Van Kruiningen, H.J., Watson, L.D., Stoke, P.E. & Lord, P.F. (1987) The influence of diet and feeding frequency on gastric function in the dog. *Journal of the American Animal Hospital Association*, **23**, 145–153.

Ware, W.A. (1992) Management of congestive heart failure. In *Essentials of Small Animal Internal Medicine*, pp. 42–77. Nelson, R.W. & Couto, C.G. (eds). Mosby, St Louis.

Westermark, E. (1980) The hereditary nature of canine pancreatic degenerative atrophy in the German shepherd dog. *Acta Veterinaria Scandinavica*, **21**, 389–394.

White, S.D. (1986) Food hypersensitivity in 30 dogs. *Journal of the American Veterinary Medical Association*, **188**, 695–698.

Wills, J.M. (1991) Dietary hypersensitivity in cats. *In Practice*, **13**, 87–93.

Wills, J.M., Sloth, C., Martin, P., Pennill, N. & Gettinby, G. (1993) A study of obese cats on a calorie controlled weight reduction programme. (in press).

Wolter, R. (1989) Dietetique du chen diabetique. *Practique Medicale et Chirurgiale de L'animal de Compagne*, **24**, 41–47.

Zimmer, J.F. (1986) Nutritional management of gastrointestinal diseases. In *Current Veterinary Therapy IX*, pp. 909–915, Kirk, R.W. (ed.). W.B. Saunders, Philadelphia.

# 5 / Anorexia, Enteral and Parenteral Feeding

## Appetite control

Appetite is controlled from a centre located in the hypothalamus. The centre maintains the animal in a state of hunger which is modified by a number of inhibitory inputs. These include inputs from higher centres, the action of hormones, the level of amino acids and glucose in the circulation, and the functional state of the digestive tract (Fig. 5.1).

Distension of the stomach or small intestine with food, the presence of high levels of amino acids and glucose in the circulation, and increased levels of gut hormones such as cholecystokinin, gastrin and bombesin all reduce appetite; the converse helps to stimulate appetite. Emotional factors including fear, excitement and changes in environment (as occur with hospitalization or boarding) will inhibit eating; their effect is mediated through the cerebral cortex. Various central neurotransmitters including catecholamines, serotonin and interleukin 1 also reduce appetite. Dopamine and opioids are thought to stimulate the appetite (Macy & Ralston, 1989).

## Anorexia/dysphagia

When a dog or cat is described as being 'off its food' a distinction must be made between the animal being anorexic or dysphagic. Dysphagia may be defined as difficulty in swallowing, aglutition or inability to swallow. Usually the animal has the desire to eat but is physically unable to do so through mechanical or neurological disorder (Table 5.1). In this situation the physical damage must be repaired before eating can occur and, while this is being carried out, nutrition must be provided by some other means. It is inappropriate to stimulate appetite in this situation as the animal has not lost the desire to eat, only the ability to eat.

Anorexia, on the other hand, may be defined as a lack of appetite, no desire to eat, a diminished appetite or an aversion to food. In these cases there is usually some systemic disease which has depressed the hunger centre in the hypothalamus. The animal has the ability to eat but has lost the desire. Pyrexia, pain, inflammation, autoimmune disease, sepsis and infection result in depressed appetite thought to be mediated through interleukin 1 which is released from mononuclear cells. Tryptophan is elevated in the serum of patients with tumours and this is thought to be the cause of anorexia in neoplastic patients (Macy & Ralston, 1989). Successful treat-

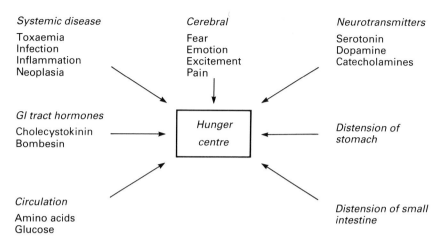

**Fig. 5.1** Factors which may affect the appetite of dogs and cats.

**Table 5.1** Conditions which may lead to dysphagia in the dog and cat

Fracture of the mandible
Palatine defects
Inflammation or infection in mouth or pharynx
Neoplasms in mouth or pharynx
Cricopharyngeal achalasia
Oesophageal disease
Myasthenia gravis
Dental disease
Myositis
Neurological defects

ment depends on specific drug therapy and efforts to stimulate the appetite.

Protein calorie malnutrition (PCM) may be defined as an inadequate intake of protein and energy resulting in a negative nitrogen and energy balance. PCM occurs when the animal is starved, anorexic, dysphagic, or has some systemic disease, infection or trauma. In these situations PCM rapidly develops, leading to progressive weight loss, immunodeficiency, anaemia, weakness, hypoproteinaemia, poor wound healing and organ failure.

The effects of starvation and true anorexia on the metabolism are different, but it is important to have an understanding of the needs of dysphagic and anorexic animals. During starvation in a normal healthy animal there is a decrease in glucose, amino acids and fatty acids absorbed from the small intestine. This results in the breakdown of hepatic glycogen stores (glycogenolysis) and formation of glucose from amino acids (gluconeogenesis) in order to maintain the blood sugar level within the normal range. This must be a rapid process as glucose is essential for the normal function of red blood cells, the CNS and kidneys. Other body systems can adapt to using other forms of energy such as fatty acids.

After a few days of starvation all the glycogen stored in the liver is used up, so gluconeogenesis becomes even more important as a source of glucose (Donaghue, 1989). Glucose cannot be produced from fatty acids and so amino acids are preferentially used (Wheeler & McGuire, 1989); this leads to increased blood ammonia levels, increased urea excretion and a negative nitrogen balance. As there is no body store of protein, all the protein used for this purpose comes from functional tissues. The net result is a loss of function of many organs, weakness and loss of lean muscle mass. Metabolic rate and physical activity are also reduced. After 7–10 days the CNS can adapt to using ketone bodies as an energy source which spares tissue protein. If this adaptation was not possible, the loss of lean muscle mass would be so rapid that death would occur within a very short time after starvation (Labato, 1990; Wheeler & McGuire, 1989).

Where the animal is anorexic because it is clinically unwell the situation is different. There is often a marked increase in metabolic rate and development of a negative nitrogen balance, with no mechanism to preserve tissue proteins. Tissues damaged, either through infection or trauma, preferentially use glucose as an energy source. The amount of glucose required is directly proportional to the degree of tissue damage present. The provision of glucose in this situation is usually not helpful as it tends to be too little to provide the calories required. It also stimulates insulin secretion which inhibits fat breakdown and stimulates further protein catabolism. In this way PCM is accelerated in sick animals, especially those which are anorexic. The rapid loss of functional protein leads to reduced organ function including: reduced cardiac output, decreased pulmonary oxygenation, and loss of mucosal integrity of the gastro-intestinal tract. The latter results in invasion of bacteria from the gut leading to sepsis which is often observed in severely ill animals in a state of PCM. This is compounded by the development of immunodeficiency also due to PCM. Cats are susceptible to even short periods of anorexia, because of their daily requirement for arginine in order to allow the conversion of ammonia to urea. Without arginine this conversion cannot occur and ammonia rapidly builds up in the circulation causing serious central nervous signs and even death.

Unfortunately there are no clinical signs or laboratory tests which are pathognomonic of PCM and the need for nutritional support. A variety of factors should be considered by the clinician when evaluating any case:

1   The presence of anorexia for >3 days.
2   The progressive loss of fat deposits and lean muscle mess; weight loss >5%.
3   The presence of hypoproteinaemia (albumin <15 g/l).
4   Severity of the infection or trauma.

5   The presence of poor wound healing.
6   Detection of a non-regenerative anaemia.
7   Development of secondary infections.

Clinically animals will be lethargic, weak and susceptible to infections. If any of the above factors are present in any individual it should be assumed that PCM is present and consideration should be given to nutritional support (Muir & Dibartola, 1983; Wheeler & McGuire, 1989).

## Appetite stimulation

In most situations the clinician will wish to restore appetite and adequate nutritional intake as rapidly as possible. Where the digestive tract is functional, then nutrition should always be provided by this route. Only when the digestive tract is not functional should parenteral (intravenous) feeding be considered. However, before resorting to the more complex methods of providing nutrition, there are several simpler methods which often stimulate appetite (Table 5.2).

Initially the state of hydration should be determined and water and electrolyte deficiencies should be corrected. If pain is suspected then analgesics should be given and efforts should be made to make the patient more comfortable. Provision of a warm, dry and stress-free environment is also a very important part of therapy.

Some animals refuse to eat because they are hospitalized, and their appetite is restored simply by sending them home. If the patient can be treated at home without compromising the treatment regime, then this

Table 5.2 Methods which may be used to stimulate appetite and provide adequate nutrition in dogs and cats. The list starts with the simplest techniques and progresses to the more complex procedures

Provide a suitable stress-free environment
Relieve pain
Rehydrate
Provide highly palatable and digestible food
Hand feed
Use of drugs:
    B vitamins
    Benzodiazepines
    Corticosteroids
    Megestrol acetate
Enteral feeding:
    Force feeding
    Orogastric tube
    Nasogastric tube
    Pharyngostomy tube
    Gastrostomy tube
Parenteral feeding

option should be considered. It will be necessary to advise the owners clearly and precisely about dietary regimes as well as other therapies. However, if the owner is considered unreliable and unlikely to provide the necessary nutritional and drug therapy, then the patient should be retained in the hospital and the initial treatment regime administered by the nursing staff.

Before the more complex methods of appetite stimulation are considered, it is important to consider the simple but often successful methods which are available. Provision of a stress-free environment together with time spent nursing and comforting the patient will often provide reassurance. Frequently food will then be accepted by hand and then from a feeding bowl.

Cats are true carnivores and tend to eat the same diet and resent dietary change. They prefer slightly acid foods and prefer food warmed to body temperature. Smell is important in the selection of food and is especially important when respiratory disease is present. Always check what the cat is normally fed and use this in the hospital, at least initially. Wide shallow feeding bowls should be used as cats do not like their whiskers touching the bowl while feeding. Petting and affection improve feeding behaviour.

Dogs tend to like sweet foods and may regulate food intake depending on the energy density of the diet, although in practise the ability to do this varies considerably. Dogs frequently select food using smell, often preferring strong smelling foods such as garlic. They also respond well to petting and affection.

Unless the diet is highly palatable and attractive to the patient this effort will be to no avail. It is pointless trying to persuade a sick animal to eat the ideally formulated veterinary diet if it is not palatable. A highly-palatable and digestible diet of generally high energy density providing the calories needed in these hypermetabolic patients should be supplied. If the patient refuses the veterinary diet of choice, then a variety of different aromatic foods should be offered. These must be fresh, and gentle heating often enhances their flavour. Frequently the patient will select one of these diets which can be used to restore appetite and slowly weaned on to a suitable veterinary diet.

Anorexic dogs and cats rapidly become deficient in the water-soluble B vitamins. This is said to further depress the appetite. For this reason B vitamins have been suggested as an appetite stimulant although their efficacy has not been proved. However, injecting B vitamins will correct any deficiency state which may be present.

Benzodiazepines have been used to stimulate appetite but their efficacy varies considerably. Diazepam works most effectively when given IV at 0.1 mg/kg. Oxazepam orally is said to be more effective in cats at 2.5 mg/cat, with the appetite being restored within 20 minutes of administration.

Benzodiazepines stimulate appetite by acting directly as an anti-serotonin agent or in a similar manner to dopamine (Macy & Ralston, 1989). Gluco-corticoids have also been used to stimulate appetite by central action on inhibitors, such as serotonin, and locally by reducing inflammation. Prednisolone at 0.25 mg/kg every second day has been used successfully to stimulate the appetite. Aspirin may stimulate the appetite by inhibition of interleukin 1 as well as by reducing fever. Megestrol acetate at 1 mg/kg/day orally inconsistently results in appetite stimulation and weight gain in some animals although the mode of action has not been determined (Macy & Ralston, 1989). Nandrolone at 5 mg/kg weekly by intramuscular injection can also stimulate appetite. When this drug works the effect tends to last longer than that produced by glucocorticoids or benzodiazepines.

Great care is required when using these drugs as they may be contra-indicated in some clinical conditions. They should only be given under direct veterinary supervision and only after simpler and often just as effec-tive methods have proved unsuccessful.

Unfortunately it is not uncommon to be faced with a patient with does not respond to these measures. In these situations it is important not to ignore their nutritional requirements but to consider the use of more complex feeding methods including enteral and parenteral techniques.

## Enteral and parenteral feeding

Nutritional support should always be considered if oral intake has been reduced for more than 3 days, where there has been significant surgical intervention leading to anorexia, or where there has been a loss of more than 5% of body weight (Armstrong & Lippert, 1988). Parenteral feeding is the term used to describe the provision of intravenous nutrients. This method should only be used where the animal is anorexic or dysphagic and where the digestive tract is not functioning (Donaghue, 1989) (Table 5.3). It might be used in conditions where there is persistent vomiting, obstruc-tion of the digestive tract, acute pancreatitis, in paralytic ileus or in the unconscious patient.

Table 5.3 Conditions where parenteral feeding methods should be considered in preference to enteral feeding

Following gastro-intestinal surgery
Repair of mandibular/maxillary fractures
Obstruction of the gastro-intestinal tract
Acute pancreatitis
Persistent vomiting
Paralytic ileus
Unconsciousness
Neurological defects in swallowing

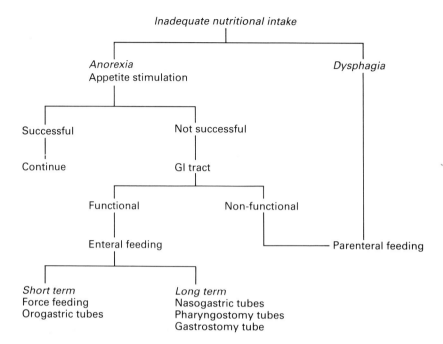

**Fig. 5.2** Method of evaluating which feeding procedure to adopt when presented with an anorexic or dysphagic dog or cat.

Enteral feeding is the term applied to the provision of nutrients introduced artificially into the digestive tract. This should always be the method of choice where the digestive tract is functioning normally. It is also easier and cheaper to carry out than parenteral feeding (Fig. 5.2). Enteral feeding usually involves the administration of nutrients either by force feeding or through a tube inserted into the digestive tract. Orogastric, pharyngostomy, nasogastric and gastrostomy tubes are the types most frequently employed.

The decision as to which type of enteral feeding to use will depend on a variety of factors including:

1   The functional capacity of the digestive tract.
2   Whether the patient is conscious or unconscious.
3   The length of time feeding is required.
4   The physical condition of the patient.
5   Patient tolerance to the procedures.
6   The ability of the patient to tolerate an anaesthetic.
7   The cost involved.

## Force feeding

This method is only suitable when the anorexic patient is conscious and not dysphagic as it requires the animal to have the ability to swallow normally.

The technique can be used in both dogs and cats but is more difficult in brachycephalic breeds. Proprietary dog or cat food may be used. Moist foods are easier to administer than dry foods but large amounts are needed to provide calorie requirements because of their high moisture content (often >70%). For this reason a canned food with a high energy density should be used.

Food may be inserted into the back of the mouth, using a syringe with the tip removed or using a preformed food bolus. The animal is then allowed to swallow normally before any further food is introduced. This method of feeding is generally poorly tolerated and patients often struggle or refuse to swallow, and may become distressed. For this reason it is not recommended except in emergency situations when no other method of feeding can be made available or when feeding is required for only 2–3 days.

## Orogastric tubes

Orogastric tubes are basically stomach tubes which are inserted via the oral cavity, passed down the oesophagus and into the stomach. They cannot be left in place but must be removed after each feeding period. They are difficult to introduce because of poor patient cooperation, especially when repeated, resulting in struggling and distress. For this reason orogastric tubes should only be used over a period of 2–3 days. There is also a risk of tracheal intubation and subsequent tissue damage or inhalation of food. Where long term enteral feeding is required one of the permanent tube placement methods should be considered in preference to this method.

## Nasogastric tubes

This type of tube is difficult to insert but once positioned may be left permanently in place until enteral feeding is no longer required. It is the tube of choice where an anaesthetic cannot be administered but long-term feeding is required. It is better tolerated than the orogastric tube. The advantage of this type of tube is that the patient may eat and drink normally with the tube in place, thus allowing the clinician to determine when normal feeding behaviour has been restored before removing the tube.

Generally, polyvinyl or thermoplastic polyurethane tubes are used, although the former tend to become hard if placed accidentally into the stomach, making removal difficult. The size of tube required depends on the species and breed involved, but usually a size 5–10 French is suitable.

The tube is placed along the side of the patient and the length required is measured from the nose to the distal oesophagus (9th to 10th rib space)

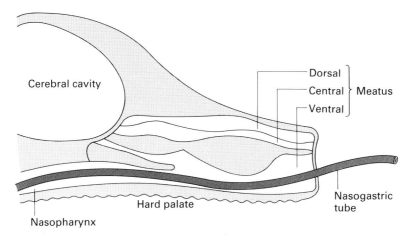

**Fig. 5.3** Correct location of a nasogastric tube in the dog using the ventral nasal meatus.

and marked on the tube. Local anaesthetic is instilled into the nasal passage and then the external nares is elevated, thus lifting the upper lip and exposing the teeth. It is then possible to insert the tube directly down into the ventral meatus taking great care not to damage the maxillary or ethmoid turbinates. Some resistance to the advancment of the tube through the ventral meatus is often encountered, but once through passage becomes easier into the pharynx (Fig. 5.3). This resistance is not encountered in cats which have a wide ventral meatus. The tube is advanced into the oesophagus as the patient swallows. By stopping at the predetermined mark the end of the tube should be at the distal oesophagus.

Ideally the position of the tube should be checked using radiography. If the tube is allowed to pass into the stomach there is a risk of reflux oesophagitis or the tube becoming hard and difficult to remove. The tube is sutured to the skin at the external nares and held in position at the back of the head by bandages. This prevents the patient removing the tube. Only liquid food can be administered using this technique, either commercially supplied or using a liquidized moist dog or cat food. Always flush the tube prior to and after feeding using sterile saline.

**Pharyngostomy tubes**

The pharyngostomy tube, like the nasogastric tube, is designed to be left in place for as long as required, and will allow the animal to eat and drink normally while in place. However, placement of the pharyngostomy tube requires a general anaesthetic and surgical intervention. Careful positioning is required to avoid the risk of entrapping the epiglottis, preventing it closing during attempts at eating and drinking. This occurs if the tube is

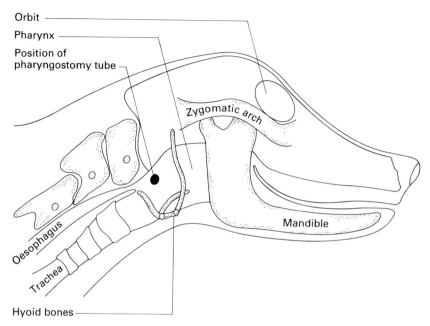

Orbit

Pharynx

Position of
pharyngostomy tube

Zygomatic arch

Oesophagus

Trachea

Mandible

Hyoid bones

**Fig. 5.4** The position for placement of a pharyngostomy tube.

placed too low in the lateral wall of the pharynx (Crowe, 1986b). For these reasons this type of tube is now less popular. Tissue swelling and haematoma formation can occur following insertion and will result in temporary inspiratory stridor.

Following induction of anaesthesia and intubation, the left side of the neck is aseptically prepared caudal to the mandible. The exact site of the incision is located using a finger inserted into the pharynx, where the hyoid bones should be felt. The finger is pushed against the lateral wall of the pharynx at its caudodorsal corner and a skin incision made at this point (Fig. 5.4). Blunt disection is carried out to make a hole into the pharynx large enough to pass the tube selected. The tube is passed through the incision into the pharynx, and using a finger the tube is guided into the oesophagus. The final position of the tube should be in the distal oesophagus. The tube is fixed using stay sutures to the skin of the neck and curved round to the back of the head.

Rubber or silicone tubes are generally used for this technique, and the size used varies considerably. Some clinicians prefer a small diameter tube (8 French) which requires the use of liquid enteral foods and is prone to blocking and kinking. Other clinicians prefer the use of larger diameter tubes (14 French) which permit the use of homogenized dog/cat food and are less likely to kink or block in use. In general, sizes 8–10 French are preferred for cats and sizes 10–14 for dogs.

Pharyngostomy tubes can be left in position for long periods of time without complication, so long as they are carefully maintained. The incision site must be kept clean using antiseptic ointments and clean dressings daily. The tube must be flushed with sterile saline after feeding and kept capped to prevent aerophagia.

Removal of the tube is carried out by releasing the stay sutures and gently pulling the tube out. The tube must be capped in case it contains food, which may be inhaled during this procedure. The skin incision, if clean, will heal within a few days of removal without suturing.

## Gastrostomy tube

In this case the tube is inserted directly into the stomach through an incision in the abdominal wall. It is useful in situations where the other tubes are not tolerated or where the use of pharyngeal or oesophageal tubes is contraindicated. Although slightly more complicated to insert, the gastrostomy tube performs very well and can be left in place for long periods of time. Like the pharyngostomy tube it requires to be inserted under general anaesthesia and with the aid of an endoscope.

Once anaesthetized, the patient is placed in right lateral recumbency and the left costal area is aseptically prepared. An endoscope is placed in the stomach and the stomach is inflated with air. The tip of the endoscope is positioned against a suitable area of the stomach wall so that the light can be seen on the outside. A stab incision is made at this site and an 14 gauge catheter inserted into the stomach. A suture is passed through the catheter and is grasped by the endoscope forceps and pulled out through the mouth. A mushroom catheter is attached to the suture and pulled down into the stomach through the incision (Lewis *et al.*, 1986). Once firmly placed

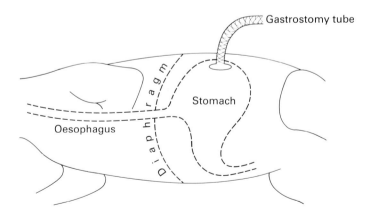

**Fig. 5.5** Diagrammatic representation of the location of a gastrostomy tube in the stomach of a dog.

against the stomach and abdominal wall, the mushroom catheter is sutured into place (Fig. 5.5). The tube should be capped to prevent air entering the stomach, and a dressing applied around the abdomen to protect the gastrostomy tube and site of incision.

Although there are few complications using this method, infection at the site of the incision is the most likely problem to occur. Unlike the other methods, removal of this catheter requires a further general anaesthetic and endoscopic retrieval of the cut end of the mushroom catheter from the stomach.

### Calculating nutritional requirements

The aim of enteral feeding is to provide all the energy, protein, vitamins and minerals required by the patient which is anorexic or dysphagic. It is important not to neglect water which is the most important nutrient and may be required together with electrolytes by many patients. In order to determine nutritional requirements the clinician must have some understanding of dog and cat nutrition. Much of this information will be found elsewhere in this book. The intention of the next section of this chapter is to discuss enteral feeding requirements of dogs and cats, and it assumes some knowledge of nutrition.

Basal energy requirement (BER) is the energy required by an animal at rest in a postabsorptive state, in a comfortable, stree-free environment at an even temperature and without disease (Armstrong & Lippert, 1988). Maintenance energy requirement (MER) is BER plus the energy needed by the animal to acquire and assimilate food; it includes physical activity, digestion and absorption of food. The BER value in kcal (1 kcal = 4.184 kJ) can be determined using the following formulae (Wheeler & McGuire, 1989):

For animals >2 kg, BER (kcal ME/day) = [30 × weight (kg)] + 70
For animals <2 kg, BER (kcal ME/day) = $70 \times$ weight $(kg)^{0.75}$

It is very difficult to determine accurately the energy needs of sick dogs and cats (Table 5.4). However, most animals in this category have an elevated metabolic rate but should not be fed high carbohydrate meals as they may have insulin insensitivity and consequent risk of hyperglycaemia.

**Table 5.4** Energy requirements for dogs and cats with various clinical conditions. Note that BER and not MER is used to calculate requirements

| | |
|---|---|
| Hospitalized dog or cat | BER × 1.3 |
| Following major trauma/surgery | BER × 1.6 |
| Neoplasia | BER × 1.6 |
| Severe infection or sepsis | BER × 1.8 |
| Major burns | BER × 2.0 |

Therefore protein and fat should be used to provide their energy requirements. Hypermetabolism may persist during the convalescent phase of up to 6 weeks (Donoghue, 1989). This occurs because the insulin:glucagon ratio is reversed, which in turn is due to the effects of growth hormone, catacholamines and cortisol produced in the stressed animal. The labile proteins most frequently utilized include muscle mass, visceral protein, collagen, albumin and immunoglobulin, which are broken down to amino acids and then converted to glucose (gluconeogenesis).

Such a protein loss results in major weight loss which can be fatal if left unchecked. Death usually occurs when the loss exceeds 45% (Crowe, 1986a). Nonetheless it is possible to make a reasonable assumption of their requirements, and a hospitalized dog or cat requires approximately 25% more calories than the normal BER. For every 1°C increase in body temperature a further increase in energy of 13% is required (Page *et al.*, 1979). Infections raise BER by up to 50% and surgery from 10 to 100%. Using this knowledge it is possible to predict the energy requirements of most individuals (Table 5.4). Great care is required with these assessments as individuals will vary considerably in their requirements. Practically the clinician should watch for sudden and rapid changes in body weight. Sudden increases in body weight may suggest fluid retention while sudden losses mean loss of lean muscle mass.

In general it is very unlikely that body weight will increase during the course of an illness, but provision of adequate calories and protein should halt any further decline in body weight and return the animal to a positive nitrogen balance.

Fats and carbohydrates may equally be used to provide energy in enteral diets. Diets with high levels of monosaccharides should be avoided as they cause a marked increase in osmotic tension in the intestine which is detrimental compared with more complex polysaccharides such as starch. However, diets rich in starch can only be effectively utilized if exocrine pancreatic function is intact. Where exocrine pancreatic function is impaired, hydrolysates of starch which contain mainly oligosaccharides may be used in place of monosaccharides and polysaccharides (Crowe, 1986c). Fats are an excellent source of energy, providing more than twice the energy content of carbohydrate or proteins. Generally, LCT are used, but this does require intact exocrine pancreatic function. If lipase is thought to be deficient MCT may be used to provide a good source of energy without the need for enzymatic digestion prior to absorption (Simpson, 1987).

No definitive information is available regarding the protein requirements of sick animals, and until nitrogen balance studies have been carried out only estimates of protein requirements can be given. It has been recommended that dogs should receive 5–7.5 g protein/100 kcal (21–31 g/100 kJ), while cats should receive 6–9 g protein/100 kcal (25–38 g/100 kJ) (Wheeler

& McGuire, 1989). Crowe (1986a) recommends 17–25% of calories as protein (4.25–6.25 g protein/100 kcal [18–26 g/100 kJ]) and for cats 20–30% of calories as protein (5–7.5 g protein/100 kcal [21–31 g/100 kJ]). These protein values should be reduced in situations where renal or hepatic failure is diagnosed to 3 g protein/100 kcal (13 g/100 kJ) for dogs and 4 g protein/100 kcal (17 g/100 kJ) for cats (Wheeler & McGuire, 1989).

All the other non-energy nutrients are also required in increased amounts due to the raised metabolic rate. Essential fatty acids, vitamins and minerals must be increased in the diet provided (Crowe, 1986a).

To calculate the energy requirements of a sick animal it is necessary to know its body weight in kilograms, the type of condition affecting the animal and the calorie density of the diet to be used. The calorie density and protein content of some veterinary diets used for enteral feeding are shown in Table 5.5. Using the data described above it is possible to calculate the energy and protein requirements of dogs and cats with various clinical conditions (Table 5.6).

Orogastric tubes may use both homogenized pet food or commercial liquid enteral diets. When nasogastric tubes are used both continuous or bolus feeding may be employed. There is less tendency to vomiting when the former is used. However even in this case a rest period of 6–8 hours is required each day. Metoclopramide can be used to reduce vomiting by IV infusion at 1 mg/kg/day. The tube must be flushed out with sterile water after each feeding, or during the rest period each day, to prevent blockage.

Gastrostomy tubes being of relatively large diameter can use homogenized pet food without difficulty. It is usual not to feed for 12 hours after inserting this tube to allow gastric motility to return to normal. Patients should be fed six to eight times daily, ensuring the tube is flushed clean and

**Table 5.5** Human and veterinary diets which may be used to supply calories and protein when enteral feeding methods are employed

| Product | Energy* | Protein |
|---|---|---|
| *Human* | | |
| Ensure (Abbott) | 106 kcal/ml | 0.037 g/ml |
| Isocal (Mead Johnson) | 104 kcal/ml | 0.034 g/ml |
| Osmolite (Abbott) | 106 kcal/ml | 0.037 g/ml |
| *Veterinary* | | |
| Hills p/d diet (dogs) | 156 kcal/100 g | 9.4 g/100 g |
| Pedigree canine concentration diet | 137 kcal/100 g | 10.8 g/100 g |
| Reanimyl (Virbac) | 90 kcal/100 g | 5.3 g/100 g |
| Hills p/d diet (cats) | 158 kcal/100 g | 15.7 g/100 g |
| Whiskas feline concentration diet | 119 kcal/100 g | 11.0 g/100 g |

* 1 kcal = 4.184 kJ.

**Table 5.6** Daily energy and protein requirements for an adult dog weighing 20 kg with a severe infection requiring enteral nutrition. The clinician decides that a homogenized commercial pet food will be used in conjunction with a pharyngostomy tube

$$BER = 30 \times 20 + 70$$
$$= 670 \, kcal \, (2803 \, kJ)$$

$$BER \times 1.8 \, (for \, infection)$$
$$= 1206 \, kcal \, (5046 \, kJ)$$

*Amount of food required to give this energy level*
The veterinary diet contains 1.48 kcal (6.19 kJ)/g of food
$$= 1206 \div 1.48$$
$$= 814.9 \, g \, of \, diet$$

Protein requirement based on 6 g protein/100 kcal
$$= 1206 \div 100 \times 6$$
$$= 72.4 \, g \, protein \, is \, required$$

The amount of protein fed in 814.9 g of diet
$$= 0.09 \times 814.9$$
$$= 73.3 \, g \, of \, protein$$

*Is a protein supplement required?*
Amount required − amount fed
$$= 72.4 - 73.3$$

A surplus of 0.9 g protein is being fed. No supplement is required in this case

capped after each feeding period. Only 25% of energy requirements should be given on the first day and the level increased slowly to 100% in no less than 4 days, unless complications arise.

The body weight of the patient should be carefully monitored and blood and urine glucose checked daily. It is not uncommon to create hyperglycaemia when enteral feeding is initiated, and if this is not corrected within 2 or 3 days the amount of calories fed should be reduced.

## Parenteral nutrition

Total parenteral nutrition (TPN) also known as parenteral hyperalimentation, describes the provision of all essential nutrients by IV administration. Many of the regimes used in dogs and cats have been adapted from human medicine and there are few solutions for parenteral nutrition specifically produced for animals. Partial parenteral nutrition (PPN) describes the administration of some essential nutrients by IV infusion, but it is possible that such administrations may still leave the patient in negative nitrogen and energy balance.

The advantages of TPN are that it allows the maintenance of nutrition in situations where the gastro-intestinal tract is not functioning. Using the

IV route ensures nutrients reach the tissues rapidly following administration and it prevents further deterioration of the patient until enteral nutrition can be restored (Muir & Dibartola, 1983). The main disadvantages are that solutions are expensive, that strict aseptic technique is required and that metabolic disturbances can occur. Many of the solutions used for TPN are hypertonic and must be administered into the vena cava or jugular veins in order to prevent thrombophlebitis (Muir & Dibartola, 1983; Labato, 1990). However, some solutions are isotonic and may be used in peripheral veins such as the cephalic vein. It is therefore very important to determine the tonicity of the solution prior to administration.

*Solutions used for TPN*

The basic components of TPN include amino acids, lipids and glucose. Non-protein calories are usually provided from fat and carbohydrate. In dogs the majority of calories are provided in equal proportions from fat and dextrose. However, more care is required with cats as they normally obtain significant calories from protein. In renal or hepatic failure the protein level for dogs and cats must be reduced.

Traditionally, dextrose solutions have been used in veterinary practice to provide energy, but unfortunately most of these solutions do not adequately meet the patient's calorie requirements. They would have to be given in very large volumes or at very rapid infusion rates to achieve the desired calorie intake. This speed of administration would almost certainly result in the development of hyperglycaemia and glycosuria (Michell *et al.*, 1989). It is therefore important to give only 25% of the calculated dextrose load on the first day and increase this slowly to the calculated volume over 3 days (Lippert & Armstrong, 1989).

Fructose, sorbitol (which is converted to fructose by the liver) and ethyl alcohol may be used in place of dextrose as they do not cause hyperglycaemia or require insulin for utilization. However, when used in large volumes they can cause lactic acidosis (Michell *et al.*, 1989).

Intralipid contains soya bean oil, egg phospholipid and glycerol. The product is available as 10% or 20% solutions giving 1100 kcal (4.6 MJ) and 2000 kcal (8.4 MJ)/l respectively. They provide a rich source of calories and essential fatty acids, in a small volume compared with dextrose solutions. Lipids should not be used in hyperlipaemic animals or those with hepatic disease and must be used with care in cats where hepatic lipidosis may develop. Unlike dextrose solutions, lipids may be given by slow but continuous infusion while monitoring serum triglyceride levels to ensure hyperlipaemia does not occur.

Protein is normally given as crystalline amino acid solutions which may also contain electrolytes. These amino acid solutions normally contain all the essential amino acids with the exception of taurine. Where TPN is to be provided for cats, then consideration of taurine requirements will have to be made. The cat requires at least 10 mg/kg/day of available taurine (Wills, 1991). Adequate levels of arginine are also essential to ensure the conversion of ammonia to urea proceeds normally (Lewis *et al.*, 1986). Aminoplex 5 (Geistlich) contains amino acids, sorbitol, ethanol and electrolytes, and provides 5 g protein and 1000 kcal (4.2 MJ)/l. The average cat would require 500 ml of this solution while a 10 kg dog would require 800 ml. This should be infused at a rate of less than 100 ml/hour into a central vein. Excess protein or amino acids can lead to depression, vomiting and convulsions, together with elevated blood urea levels (Michell *et al.*, 1989).

**Table 5.7** Method of calculating the total parenteral nutritional requirements of protein, carbohydrates and lipids for dogs and cats

---

BER = 30 × weight (kg) + 70
    = $x$ kcal/day

Requirements during illness, see Table 5.4

Protein requirement:
    By an adult dog  = 4 g/kg
    PLE or burns    = 6 g/kg
    Renal/hepatic
       failure      = 1.5 g/kg
    Protein required = $y$ g/day

Volume of protein solution required using 5% aminoplex
(5% = 50 g/ml)
Volume required = $y$ g protein/day ÷ 50
               = $v$ ml of protein solution for infusion

Protein calories = 4 kcal/g protein
           = $y$ g protein × 4
           = $p$ kcal from protein

Total kcal/day required ($x$) − kcal from protein ($p$) = kcal from carbohydrate and fat
Normally give remaining calories in a 50:50 ratio of lipid:carbohydrate

50% from carbohydrates = $a$ kcal
Therefore using 40% dextrose giving 1.7 kcal/ml
ml of solution required = 50% of kcal ÷ 1.7
                   = $c$ ml of 40% dextrose

50% from lipids = $b$ kcal
Therefore using 20% intralipid giving 2 kcal/ml
ml of solution required = 50% kcal ÷ 2
                   = $l$ ml of 20% intralipid

Total volume for infusion = $v + c + l$

Ensure weekly injections of multi-vitamin preparation

---

1 kcal = 4.184 kJ

Electrolytes are normally provided with the amino acid solutions. Vitamins are usually provided as multi-vitamin preparations given by injection or infused with other solutions. Care should always be taken to ensure the patient is adequately hydrated prior to administration of TPN.

Calculation of the protein and calorie requirements of a hospitalized animal for TPN may be determined in exactly the same manner as that used for enteral nutrition. Once the BER and stress factor has been calculated for the individual concerned, it is then possible to determine the amount of protein and calories required and thus the volume of each solution required (Table 5.7).

*Administration of solutions*

When several different solutions are to be given it is practically useful if the solutions can be mixed and given through the same catheter. However, care is required to ensure the solutions are compatible and the instructions accompanying each solution should be read carefully to ensure they can be safely mixed.

Great care is required when administering these solutions as they provide ideal media for bacterial growth. A sterile catheter must always be used along with strict aseptic technique when handling the catheter and solutions. Peristaltic pumps are useful for ensuring that solutions are given at the correct rate and over the correct period of time. During the first day of administration only 25% of the computed dextrose volume should be given and the response to this administration monitored. If hyperglycaemia and glycosuria do not develop then the amount given can be increased to the total computed volume over the next 2 days.

*Monitoring response to TPN*

It is important to monitor the response to therapy very carefully. The complications which may occur while using TPN include the following:
1   Mechanical occlusion of the catheter.
2   Infection at the site of the catheter or within the catheter.

**Table 5.8** Monitoring requirements for various physiological parameters

| | |
|---|---|
| Temperature, pulse, respiration | Three times daily |
| Urine glucose | Twice daily |
| Body weight | Daily |
| PCV | Daily |
| Triglyceride | Daily |
| Sodium, potassium, calcium, phosphorus | Daily |
| Routine haematology | Weekly |

**3** Thrombophlebitis, especially if peripheral vessels are used.

**4** Hyperglycaemia and gylcosuria through rapid dextrose infusions.

**5** Hypokalaemia through intracellular movement of potassium and glucose.

**6** High blood urea where excessive protein infusions are given.

**7** Hyperlipaemia where excess lipid is infused.

From the complications outlined above the clinician can appreciate the need for careful monitoring. For this reason the parameters in Table 5.8 should be checked routinely.

## References

Armstrong, P.J. & Lippert, A.C. (1988) Selected aspects of enteral and parenteral nutritional support. *Seminars in Veterinary Medicine and Surgery*, **3**, 216–226.

Crowe, D.T. (1986a) Enteral nutrition for critically ill or injured patients – part I. *Compendium of Continuing Education for the Practicing Veterinarian*, **8**, 603–612.

Crowe, D.T. (1986b) Enteral nutrition for critically ill or injured patients – part II. *Compendium of Continuing Education for the Practicing Veterinarian*, **8**, 719–732.

Crowe, D.T. (1986c) Enteral nutrition for critically ill or injured patients – part III. *Compendium of Continuing Education for the Practicing Veterinarian*, **8**, 826–838.

Donoghue, S. (1989) Nutritional support of hospitalised patients. *Veterinary Clinics of North America: Small Animal Practice*, **19**, 475–495.

Labato, M.A. (1990) Nutritional intervention. *Pet Veterinarian*, **5**, 31–35.

Lewis, L.D., Morris, M.L. & Hand, M.S. (1987) Anorexia, inition, and critical care nutrition. In *Small Animal Clinical Nutrition III*, pp. 5.1–5.43, Mark Morris Associates, Kansas.

Lippert, A.C. & Armstrong, P.J. (1989) Parenteral nutritional support. In *Current Veterinary Therapy X*, pp. 25–29, Kirk, R.W. (ed.). W.B. Saunders, Philadelphia.

Macy, D. & Ralston, S.L. (1989) Cause and control of decreased appetite. In *Current Veterinary Therapy X*, pp. 18–24, Kirk, R.W. (ed.). W.B. Saunders, Philadelphia.

Michell, A.R., Bywater, R.J., Clarke, K.W., Hall, L.W. & Waterman, A.E. (1989) Metabolic and endocrine disturbances; parenteral nutrition. In *Veterinary Fluid Therapy*, pp. 222–245. Blackwell Scientific Publications, Oxford.

Muir, W.W. & Dibartola, S.P. (1983) Fluid therapy. In *Current Veterinary Therapy VIII*, pp. 28–40, Kirk, R.W. (ed.). W.B. Saunders, Philadelphia.

Page, C.P., Carlton, P.K., Andrassy, R.J., Feldtman, R.W. & Shield, C.F. (1979) Safe, cost effective post operative nutrition. Defined formula diet via needle-catheter jejunostomy. *American Journal of Surgery*, **138**, 939–945.

Simpson, J.W. (1987) Fat absorption in dogs and its diagnostic value in exocrine pancreatic insufficiency and malabsorption. In *The Veterinary Annual*, pp. 319–323, Grunsell, C.S.G., Hill, F.W.G. & Raw, M.E. (eds). Scientechnica, Bristol.

Wheeler, S.L. & McGuire, B.H. (1989) Enteral nutritional support. In *Current Veterinary Therapy X*, pp. 30–37. W.B. Saunders, Philadelphia.

Wills, J. (1991) Clam juice as a source of taurine. *Journal of Small Animal Practice*, **32**, 540.

# 6 / Nutrition and Old Age

The onset and development of old age in dogs and cats is less well-defined than the period of puppyhood or kittenhood. Puppies and kittens are readily identified by their behaviour, their size and their needs for special care. They are *expected* to be more trouble than adult animals and advice is often sought from veterinarians on vaccination, worming, training, diet and general health care. Once this period has passed, the behaviour, appearance and needs of the mature adult animal stabilize, and a pattern of life is established in which feeding and management are much the same from year to year. The onset of old age towards the end of this period is a slow process and many owners do not recognize that their pet is old until there are quite obvious indicators of ageing such as appearance, exercise intolerance, or age-related disease. The needs of dogs and cats when they are old are, nevertheless, as worthy of special consideration as when they are very young.

## Individual and breed/size variation in the onset of old age

Individual differences in the onset of the signs of old age in dogs are accentuated by size and breed differences (Table 6.1). A survey in the USA (Goldston, 1989) of the relationship between body weight and the onset of old age-related disease confirms the generally accepted view that large and giant dogs become geriatric at an earlier age than small and medium dogs (which are similar to cats).

Although there is no comparable study in other countries, data from UK sources confirms that the average life span of the giant breeds is shorter than that of other breeds (Anderson, 1990).

## Biological consequences of ageing

Veterinary care of ageing animals is dependent on a working knowledge of the underlying biological events associated with the ageing process. Although some of the published work on veterinary geriatrics is based on extrapolation of the age-related changes in man, there is a growing volume of veterinary knowledge based on experimental induction of functional deficiencies associated with ageing in dogs and cats (such as renal insufficiency), or on published clinical observations from veterinarians with a particular interest in certain age-related diseases.

**Table 6.1** Age at which dogs in various weight groups, and cats, were considered to be 'geriatric' (from Goldston, 1989)

| Category | Body weight (kg) | Age of onset |
|---|---|---|
| *Dogs* | | |
| Small | <9.1 | 11.48 ± 1.86 |
| Medium | 9.1–22.7 | 10.19 ± 1.56 |
| Large | 22.8–40.1 | 8.85 ± 1.38 |
| Giant | >40.1 | 7.46 ± 1.27 |
| *Cats* | | 11.88 ± 1.94 |

**Tissue structure and composition**

The overt changes in body structure and function, such as reduction in muscle mass, loss of skin elasticity, increased body fat, reduced physical activity and impaired homeostatic mechanisms are related to underlying cellular changes (Harman, 1981). Cell changes occur rapidly during growth and development. After maturity the rate of change is dependent on the genetic programming of individual cells or cell groups and other factors such as the accumulation of waste products, enzyme increase or depletion, and damage by free oxygen radicals. Ageing theory implicates functional changes in suppressor or helper T lymphocytes, increased auto-antibody production and decreased sensitivity of the immune system. Many of these changes appear to occur in association with ageing in all mammalian species, but because of the protected domestic environment enjoyed by dogs and cats, they become more advanced in these species than in the wild or in animals kept for production or performance. In the wild, the reduction in function which occurs in association with ageing clearly has a more detrimental effect on the life expectancy of predator or prey animals, since they are much more dependent on their physical fitness for survival than are the more protected companion animals.

**Metabolic change**

The rate of metabolism is greatest in very young and lowest in aged animals, with a long intermediate and relatively stable rate during mature adult life. In old age there is a reduced rate and efficiency of drug metabolism and reduced responsiveness to changing environmental temperature and dehydration. Although the occurrence and explanation of these changes are not well documented in old dogs and cats, they should be taken into account when assessing their clinical state and treatment. The fact that an old dog spends much of the day sleeping and seems to have a poor appetite may have less clinical significance than the same history in a younger animal, but the temptation to dump a range of potentially significant clinical signs into the 'just old age' basket should be resisted, since it may do a disservice to an old animal whose condition may be due, at least in part, to treatable disease. Some old animals are less able to recognise or respond to hot conditions by moving to a cooler place and may require to be shaded or moved to avoid heat stroke or dehydration.

The functional integrity and responsiveness of the immune system also has a part to play in the old animal's state of health and survivability. Impaired immune competence may, for instance, reduce the response of old dogs to vaccination and may underlie their increased susceptibility to neoplasia or auto-immune disease.

Both owner and veterinarian must recognize the need to manage old animals as a special category of the population with general as well as specific requirements which differ from both the young and the mature animals.

### Cardiovascular changes

In man, cardiovascular disease is probably the best known concomitant of old age, primarily because of the prevalence of acute coronary heart disease in Western populations. Reduced heart function is also a common subjective symptom among the elderly, thus increasing its prominence among age-related diseases. Cardiopulmonary disease is common in geriatric dogs, estimated at 25% incidence in dogs between 9 and 12 years and 33% in dogs of 13 years and over (Harris & Knauer, 1973).

Reduced cardiac output has widespread metabolic consequences. Cellular hypoxia results in further weakening of cardiac muscle, reduced respiratory efficiency and increased susceptibility to respiratory infection. Age-related degenerative changes are accelerated by tissue hypoxia in virtually all organs of the body; thus the onset of cardiac dysfunction may well precipitate clinical signs associated with failure of other systems which were previously maintaining an adequate performance, e.g. renal homeostasis. Andersen (1970a) noted that, despite the prevalence of heart lesions at autopsy of aged laboratory beagles, the primary cause of death was usually from causes other than heart failure.

### Toxins

Increased production and impaired elimination of endogenous toxins may be significant factors in age-related malaise. In both dogs and cats periodontal disease is an important contributor to this toxaemia (Beard & Beard, 1989). Reduced functional salivary tissue and salivary flow, possibly associated with diet, contribute to the deposition of dental calculi, chronic periodontitis and loosening followed by loss of teeth. Production and absorption of bacterial toxins and periodic bacteraemia cause or exacerbate conditions such as endocarditis and nephritis. In addition to these specific disease entities however, the normal wear and tear of the teeth may affect ingestion and selection of food. Stone- and stick-carrying dogs may show marked attrition of enamel and loss of tooth substance in their later years and this, together with malocclusions, may contribute to a predisposition to periodontal disease and its metabolic consequences.

### Urological disease

As kidneys age, their reserve capacity diminishes. Heart failure can precipitate ischaemic renal failure if cardiac function is not restored. Other reversible conditions which may, if not treated, provoke renal failure are urinary tract obstructions and infections or diabetes mellitus. The older the animal, in general, the more likely it is that the reserve capacity of the renal tissue will be overwhelmed (Krawieg, 1989).

The role of dietary protein intake in the aetiology of renal failure is unproven. There is no doubt that high levels of protein in the diet affect renal function by causing glomerular hyperfiltration, and there is evidence in man that proteinuria is commoner among meat eaters than vegetarians (Wiseman *et al.*, 1987). Although it has been shown that high dietary intakes may have a significant effect on the progression of renal failure in dogs with experimentally reduced renal function, the long-term effect of protein intake on renal function in normal dogs is less clear. In view of the naturally high protein intake of carnivorous animals, one would not have anticipated protein intake *per se* to have had a significant effect on the onset of renal failure in healthy dogs.

### Special senses

A reduction in aural and visual acuity frequently accompanies old age. Actual failure of sight or hearing has to be distinguished from an indifference to visual and aural stimuli. The onset of senile cataract rises rapidly from 12 or 13 years onwards (Fischer, 1989), but these effects are exacerbated, as in many other age-related diseases, by the fact that the long-term effects of pre-existing disease have more time to develop since dogs and cats live longer than in the past. Loss of aural acuity may only become apparent in dogs when vision has begun to deteriorate as well, since visual awareness may have been able to 'cover up' for loss of hearing.

### Skin

Skin and hair changes are often the most obvious indicators of advancing age. The coat loses its gloss, the skin becomes dry and inelastic, and there may be hair loss and depigmentation. Skin cysts and tumours become more frequent and parasitism may also become more likely.

The general loss of coat condition is probably due in part to reduction in self-grooming, but also to reduced skin circulation and secretions. Loss of skin elasticity is associated with increased calcium content and pseudo-elastin in the elastic fibres. Greying hair, particularly in the muzzle region, is particularly noticeable in dogs such as black Labrador retrievers and border collies due to the contrast with the normal black pigmentation of the hair. Reduced activity is associated with claw overgrowth and increased brittleness.

Much can be done to improve the quality of life and health of old dogs and cats by regular grooming and attention to claw length.

### Reproductive system

There is relatively little quantified data on the effects of ageing on the reproductive systems of dogs and cats. Intact bitches continue to show physiological and behavioural signs of sexual activity, though the length of the oestrus cycle increases with advancing age due, primarily, to prolongation of anoestrus (Andersen, 1970b).

## Nutrition of old dogs and cats

There are few quantitative nutritional studies on healthy old dogs and there are no specific quantitative recommendations for their nutritional requirements. The studies which have been carried out have shown that under experimental conditions old dogs made as efficient or more efficient use of dietary nutrients as young dogs (Lloyd & McCay, 1955; Sheffy *et al.*, 1985; Buffington *et al.*, 1989). On the evidence of these studies, one might conclude that there is little need for special diets for old dogs, which are apparently able to digest the essential nutrients from their food as well as or better than young dogs under the same conditions. Unlike some other biological functions, digestive efficiency has not been shown to diminish as age increases, so healthy old dogs appear to be as likely to meet their nutrient needs from a given diet as are young dogs.

Ageing has however, been described as the progressive accumulation of changes with time associated with or responsible for increasing susceptibility to disease and death. There is therefore a relatively increased likelihood that an old dog or cat will be presented for veterinary treatment, not because it is old, but because it is showing signs of some disease which, because of its age, it has contracted or which has progressed to the stage of affecting its bodily functions and quality of life. Under such circumstances, dietary advice may be appropriate and beneficial.

## Energy balance

*Obesity*

Ageing is accompanied by a progressive decrease in lean body mass and an increase in body fat with a change in its distribution. Old dogs show a decrease in basal metabolic rate and a lowering of glucose tolerance (Sheffy *et al.*, 1985). If, in addition, the amount of physical exercise given to, or taken by old dogs decreases and there is no parallel decrease in the food provided or consumed, obesity is inevitable.

The ill effects of obesity are described elsewhere (p. 86). In old dogs obesity may be even more debilitating than in younger animals due to the additional strain on systems which already have reduced capacity due to the biological effects of ageing and possible progression of chronic disease.

The successful treatment of obesity in old dogs and cats may be of even greater benefit (though more difficult) than in younger animals. The difficulty arises from the set habits and behaviour which have developed over many years in both pet and owner, the fact that the owner has become accustomed to the animal in its obese state so may lack the motivation to change it and because, as a result of the slower rate of metabolism, it takes longer to 'burn off' the excess energy stored as body fat.

Explanation to the owner of the causes and consequences of obesity is essential. The fact that obesity is both reducing the quality of life and threatening its continuation must be put over with conviction and effectiveness, using specific examples, such as impaired thermoregulation, added strain on an ageing cardiovascular system and increased pain on arthritic joints (problems with which some owners may well identify). The weight-reducing regime advised may differ from that for younger obese subjects for the following reasons:

1   Both the animal and its owner may be more resistant to fundamental dietary change because of the long habituation to the existing diet.

2   The underlying deterioration in other regulatory systems will be more advanced and thus more vulnerable to imposed metabolic change than in younger animals.

3   The option of hospitalization and radical reduction in food intake is inappropriate, since such treatment may well be less tolerable for an old animal both physiologically and psychologically than for a younger one.

4   The owner may, not unreasonably, argue that with a relatively short life expectancy anyway, they would prefer their pet to die fat and happy rather than lean and miserable!

*Dietary recommendations.* Details of the existing diet must be extracted from the owner – frequency, quantity, constituents and extra titbits. If the diet appears unbalanced nutritionally, the opportunity should be taken to correct it. Thereafter, the objective is to reduce both the energy content and the quantity fed. With the proviso that weight reduction may take longer in old obese animals than in younger ones the dietary regime described in Chapter 4 should be followed.

*Exercise.* The role of exercise in reducing obesity in old dogs should not be discounted. A reduction in energy expenditure due to changing family circumstances (children growing up and leaving home) may well have contributed to the development of the animal's obesity, so the question has to be asked whether some re-instatement of daily exercise may not benefit the animal and its owner. Clearly their general state of health must be equal to the task and any sudden increase avoided. If circumstances are not suitable to the owner's personal involvement, it is often possible to find a willing youngster in the neighbourhood who will act as an exerciser.

*Weight loss*

As in younger animals, weight loss in aged dogs and cats may be associated with the underlying disease. Periodontitis is one such condition, the prevalence of which increases with age. The effective treatment of the disease reduces the inflammation, pain and toxaemia from infected gums, all of which contribute to reduced food intake and weight loss. Provision of palatable, chewable foods, proprietary chews or marrow bones provides the jaw, tooth and gum with exercise which helps to control periodontal disease in dogs. Access to dry foods, as well as the opportunity to catch and consume prey, are probably the best preventive for cats.

Weight loss may, however, occur in old dogs without apparent underlying disease. Loss of muscle tone and volume due to diminished activity is a common feature of ageing. This may respond to improving the palatability of the diet and increasing the frequency of feeding. Palatability can be increased by warming the food and improving the protein quality. Unless the total protein content is low, it is probably unwise to increase intake in order to spare the load on the ageing kidneys.

*Thermoregulation*

The impaired ability to thermoregulate in extremes of cold and heat may require special management in old dogs and cats. Where hair loss has occurred, their defences against cold are weakened and, for dogs at least, the use of a protective overcoat during winter may be appropriate. These coats should be kept dry and clean to reduce the likelihood of acting as a reservoir for external parasites. To deny an old, sparsely-covered dog its daily walk because of cold weather may abolish one of the day's highlights, so protective covering is a sensible precaution.

In hot, sunny weather, a shaded place should always be available for dogs and cats outside – if they do not spontaneously seek it, they can be put in it. Water should always be accessible, since panting and poor renal concentrating ability are both likely to provoke dehydration which, in conjunction with diminished cardiac function, can be life-threatening.

The intake of food causes an increase in heat production the specific dynamic action (SDA) of the food. The SDA is dependent on the nature of the food. Foods rich in protein cause a much greater increase in heat output (or have a greater SDA) than carbohydrate-rich foods for any given energy intake. The main cause of the increase in heat output, which occurs within minutes of the end of a meal, is partly the increased metabolic activity of the digestive glands of the gastro-intestinal tract, but mainly the metabolism of amino acids in the liver. The chemical energy in nutrients must be transferred and stored in high energy phosphate bonds (ATP) before it becomes directly available to the tissues. Waste energy is given off as heat, which is greater when ATP is being formed as a result of the breakdown of amino acids, than when carbohydrate or fatty acid is used. For obese, old dogs in warm weather it is therefore logical to:

1   Reduce the total amount fed at each meal (to reduce SDA and obesity).
2   Feed the reduced amount in two meals rather than at a single meal.
3   Reduce the proportion of meat in a meat/biscuit mix.
4   Ensure that shade and water are always available.
5   If heat prostration does occur, remove to a cool, darkened room and wrap in wet towels.

**Protein**

No special protein needs have been demonstrated for healthy old dogs and the role of dietary protein in the causation of degenerative changes in the kidneys of dogs or cats is unproven. Increased dietary protein intake is known to increase the rate of glomerular filtration in the normal kidney and will also increase the filtration volume in partially nephrectomized dogs.

Renal damage may occur due to a wide range of causes (infectious, toxic, neoplastic, congenital and immunological) and the development and control of the consequent renal damage is described in Chapter 4. Apart from congenital disorders of the kidney, which are most likely to become manifest in young or young adult animals, most of the other effects are likely to have a progressive effect on renal function with advancing age. Even if the original lesion is not progressive, the remaining functional renal tissue reduces in amount as the animal ages and the likelihood of renal failure being precipitated by a dietary or other insult is increased.

It is unrealistic to propose some arbitrary level of protein intake for old dogs with a reduced renal reserve capacity. As proposed elsewhere (Chapter 4), the protein status of individual animals must be assessed before rational advice on protein intake can be given; a balance between the excess protein loss due to damaged glomeruli and the excess retention of the end products of metabolism due to decreased filtration and tubular function is the goal.

There is, however, good reason to advise that protein of high biological quality should provide the main source of nitrogen and amino acids so that, for any given nitrogen intake, the excretory end-products of protein metabolism are minimized, thus reducing the renal excretory load. There is a further benefit in that proteins of high biological quality, in general, improve the palatability and digestibility of the diet.

## Fat

The amount of fat in the diet can be manipulated over a wide range to control both energy intake and palatability. Where obesity is a primary problem, reduction in the dietary fat intake is an effective way of introducing negative energy balance and loss of stored body fat. Proprietary pet foods, however, contain relatively small percentages of fat, so it is important that household scraps, which are often high in fat, are eliminated from the diet. Conversely, for an old dog which is thin due to low food intake, the addition of fat to the diet has a useful role in decreasing or reversing the weight loss.

Supplementation with essential fatty acids may have a beneficial effect in old dogs with dry skins, poor coat condition and hair loss. Vegetable oils, such as corn, sunflower and olive oils, provide good sources of essential fatty acids and are readily available. They may also be administered as proprietary capsules (Efavet, Bimeda UK Ltd).

If the dietary fat level is significantly increased over a prolonged period, the intake of other nutrients may be reduced. It is important to ensure that adequate vitamin and mineral status is maintained, either by ensuring sufficient intake of a balanced diet or providing a multi-vitamin/mineral supplement.

Because of its role as a vehicle for the fat-soluble vitamins, the need to meet the minimum requirements of the essential fatty acids, and its palatability benefits, the fat content of the diet should not be less than 5% on a dry weight basis.

## Carbohydrate

Although carbohydrate is not an essential nutrient, it is nevertheless a useful and readily digestible source of energy for old dogs and cats. There is, therefore, no good reason to change the proportion of carbohydrate from that normally fed (p. 21) unless there are specific underlying disease problems such as obesity (p. 86) or diabetes mellitus (p. 82).

### Fibre

Less is known about the dietary fibre needs of dogs and cats than man. The vegetable fibre which occurs in the cereals of dry foods and mixers plays a useful role in the maintenance of faeces consistency and bowel function. Where constipation occurs in old dogs in association with diet or lack of exercise, the introduction of increased fibre in the diet (once the initial constipation has been relieved) is worth trying in order to promote normal bowel function and evacuation of the colon. Wheat bran can be added to the normal diet (although it may reduce palatability), or one of the various proprietary high-fibre diets can be substituted in part for the existing diet.

### Vitamins

The use of vitamin supplements is controversial. The argument against supplementation is that a food or diet which is 'complete and balanced' already contains all the required nutrients in the correct balance and the nutrient status can at best be unimproved by supplementary vitamins and at worst may be unbalanced.

In the case of old dogs and cats, however, there is a counter argument. Commercial diets are formulated to provide adequate levels of nutrients per unit of energy in the diet, the assumption being that the bigger the animal the greater the energy expenditure, the greater the energy (food) intake and thus the greater the nutrient intake. This is a sound and practicable arrangement, so long as energy expenditure and food intake are maintained at the 'average' or estimated levels used in the formulation of compound foods for dogs and cats. We have, however, seen that intake may be reduced voluntarily in old age or be restricted as part of a weight control regime. With any such overall reduction in food intake, there is obviously a proportional reduction in the intake of individual nutrients and, depending on the margins of each nutrient over the minimum requirement, daily intake may be reduced to levels bordering on insufficiency in old dogs.

There is little or no quantitative evidence for or against vitamin supplementation of old dogs. Previous studies (Lloyd & McCay, 1955; Sheffy et al., 1985) included no dietary vitamin data, although Sheffy et al. (1985) found no difference in the vitamin C and E status of their young and old dogs using serum assays and tests. The need for vitamin supplementation of old dogs or cats is, therefore, unproven. One may, however, advocate their use on the following grounds:

1   There is a psychological benefit to the owner (and possibly the animal) if a palatable and nutritious supplement is included in the daily regime, either given at meal times or at another regular occasion. The owner can be assured that a regular vitamin supplement may well have a health benefit for an old animal.

2   There may be a real nutritional requirement, particularly in old animals with markedly reduced food intake.

3   Appetite may be stimulated by giving a vitamin supplement shortly before the meal.

*Which vitamins?*

*Fat-soluble (A, D, E and K).* The capacity to store vitamin A in the liver and kidneys is probably reduced by age-associated changes in these organs. If dietary vitamin A intake is reduced due to dietary insufficiency or decreased food intake, body reserves of vitamin A in old dogs and cats are likely to be more quickly exhausted than in younger animals. To a lesser extent the capacity to store the other fat-soluble vitamins may also be reduced and animals become less able to rely on body stores and more dependent on a regular dietary intake either from foods known to be rich in vitamins or from fat-soluble vitamin supplements.

Whether or not dietary supplementation of these vitamins is advised depends on a clinical and nutritional evaluation. If supplementation is advised, then the importance of moderation must be stressed since, particularly for the fat-soluble vitamins, the old animal not only has limited storage capacity, but may be less resistant to overdosage.

*Water-soluble (B complex and C).* The requirements for the water-soluble vitamins of the B complex are not accurately known for dogs and cats, but the best available estimates are contained in the respective publications for the nutrient requirements of dogs (National Research Council, 1985) and cats (National Research Council, 1986). There is little or no clinical evidence that old dogs have greater requirements for these vitamins than are recommended for maintenance. Therefore, where the intake of a complete and balanced ration is normal no supplementation with B vitamins should be necessary. However, as with the fat-soluble vitamins, an old dog or cat with a substantially decreased intake of its daily ration will be closer to the minimum requirements for its body weight than an adult with a normal food intake. There is, therefore, a sound rationale for their use on a daily or more occasional basis as part of the old animal's special regime for maintaining condition and appetite, and delaying the degenerative processes of old age. Because excess requirements of B vitamins are not stored in the body, old dogs and cats are not at increased risk of overdosage.

Dogs and cats have no requirement for a dietary source of vitamin C. Occasional claims have been made, nevertheless, for a beneficial effect in specific and non-specific clinical situations. Vitamin C can be used as a urinary acidifier and is virtually non-toxic. Its value for old dogs or cats must, however, be speculative.

**Minerals**

There is no rationale for increasing the mineral intake of old dogs receiving diets in which mineral levels are adequate for maintenance. There may, however, be good reason to feed diets which are low in phosphorus to reduce the osteodystrophy and nephrocalcinosis associated with renal insufficiency. Veterinary diets are available in which phosphorus levels are low, and the antacids aluminium hydroxide or carbonate, which bind phosphorus, may also be used in conjunction with these low-phosphorus diets. Reduction in the phosphorus content of home-made diets can be achieved by substituting calcium carbonate for high phosphate bone flour or fish meal in the mineral supplement and using white bread or cooked rice as a carbohydrate source instead of cereal.

The role of dietary salt in the aetiology of cardiovascular disease in dogs and cats is unproven. Many proprietary foods provide salt levels substantially greater than minimum requirements but dogs are well able to excrete large amounts of dietary salt via the kidneys. In old animals, the problem of introducing low-salt diets for cardiac insufficiency may be greater than in younger animals, due to the fixed dietary habits which are associated with old age and the reluctance to accept a new type of food. The effect of salt itself on palatability is less important than in the human diet. Dogs are quite willing to consume unsalted meat for instance, whereas man usually finds it necessary to add salt for maximum palatability. The total avoidance of table scraps (high in salt) is essential if a low salt intake is to be achieved.

## Summary

Old age is characterized by a diminished capacity to respond to environmental challenge. Old animals, therefore have special needs which differ from other age categories. These needs include protection from extremes of heat, cold and dehydration, and increased attention to dental health and coat condition.

Digestive efficiency in dogs does not appear to be impaired by old age *per se* but obesity, weight loss or constipation, when they occur, may require more prolonged and determined treatment than in younger animals.

Reduced metabolic rate is associated with reduced food intake. Moderate supplementation by general vitamin/mineral supplements is therefore justifiable in order to maintain intake of these nutrients at recommended levels.

Although the various degenerative conditions associated with old age are often progressive, much can be done to prevent or delay their onset. The decrease in morbidity due to infectious disease and the longer life expectancy due to improved nutrition and management have resulted in an increasing proportion of the pet population which can be characterized as old. Their quality of life is dependent on the sympathetic understanding of their special needs by their owners under the professional guidance of their veterinarians.

## References

Andersen, A.C. (1970a) General pathology. In *The Beagle as an Experimental Dog*, pp. 520–546, Andersen, A.C. (ed.). Iowa State University Press, Iowa.

Andersen, A.C. (1970b) Reproduction. In *The Beagle as an Experimental Dog*, pp. 31–39, Andersen, A.C. (ed.). Iowa State University Press, Iowa.

Anderson, R.S. (1990) Age distribution in dogs and its relationship to life expectancy. *Proceedings of the 4th Nordic Symposium on Small Animal Disease*, pp. 59–61. Stockholm.

Beard, G.B. & Beard, D.M. (1989) Geriatric dentistry. *Veterinary Clinics of North America: Small Animal Practice*, **19**, 49–74.

Buffington, C.A., Branam, J.E. & Dunn, G.C. (1989) Lack of effect of age on digestibility of protein, fat and dry matter in beagle dogs (Abstract). In *Waltham Symposium No. 7. Nutrition of the Dog and Cat*, p. 397, Burger, I.H. & Rivers, J.P.W. (eds). Cambridge University Press, Cambridge.

Fischer, C.A. (1989) Geriatric ophthalmology. *Veterinary Clinics of North America: Small Animal Practice*, **19**, 103–124.

Goldston, R.T. (1989) Geriatrics and gerontology (Preface). *Veterinary Clinics of North America: Small Animal Practice*, **19**, ix–x.

Harman, D. (1981) The ageing process. *Proceedings of the National Academy of Sciences of the USA*, **78**, 7124–7128.

Harris, S.G. & Knauer, K.W. (1973) Diagnosis and treatment of common heart diseases. *Proceedings of the 40th Annual Meeting of the American Animal Hospital Association*, pp. 76–83. American Animal Hospital Association, Indiana.

Krawiec, D.R. (1989) Urologic disorders of the geriatric dog. *Veterinary Clinics of North America: Small Animal Practice*, **19**, 75–85.

Lloyd, L.E. & McCay, C.M. (1955) The utilization of nutrients by dogs of different ages. *Journal of Gerontology*, **10**, 182–187.

National Research Council (1985) *Nutrient Requirements of Dogs*. National Academy Press, Washington, DC.

National Research Council (1986) *Nutrient Requirements of Cats*. National Academy Press, Washington, DC.

Sheffy, B.E., Williams, A.J., Zimmer, J.F. & Ryan, G.D. (1985) Nutrition and metabolism of the geriatric dog. *Cornell Veterinarian*, **75**, 324–347.

Wiseman, M.J., Hunt, R., Goodwin, J.L., Keen, H. & Viberti, G.C. (1987) Dietary composition and renal function in healthy human subjects. *Nephron*, **46**, 37–42.

## Further reading

Bush, B.M. (1989) Geriatric nursing. In *Jones's Animal Nursing*, 5th edn, pp. 392–397, Lane, D.R. (ed.). Pergamon Press, Oxford.

Goldston, R.T. (ed.) (1989) Geriatrics and gerontology. *Veterinary Clinics of North America: Small Animal Practice*, **19**, 1–202.

Lewis, L.D., Morris, M.L. & Hand, M.S. (1987) Feeding the aged dog or cat. In *Small Animal Clinical Nutrition III*, pp. 3.22–3.25. Mark Morris Associates, Kansas.

Mosier, J.E. (1989) Effect of ageing on body systems of the dog. *Veterinary Clinics of North America: Small Animal Practice*, **19**, 1–12.

Mosier, J.E. (1990) Caring for the ageing dog in today's practice. *Veterinary Medicine*, **85**, 460–471.

# Appendix 1: Breeds of Dog

The following table provides information on the size and weight for different breeds of dog. It has been produced with the kind permission of Mr J. M. Evans MRCVS, editor of *Henston Vade Mecum* (small animal edn) 1992–93.

Key: H, hound; WD, working dog; UB, utility breed; NS, not specified; TER, terrier; TB, toy breed; GD, gun dog.
Conversions: 1 cm = 0.39 inches, 1 kg = 2.2 pounds.

| Breed | Class | Average height at shoulder (cm) | | Average weight of adult (kg) | | Colour/markings |
|---|---|---|---|---|---|---|
| | | Male | Female | Male | Female | |
| Affenpinscher | TB | 25.5 | 23 | 4 | 3 | Black |
| Afghan hound | H | 71 | 66 | 27 | 22.5 | Any |
| Airedale terrier | TER | 59.5 | 57 | 21.5 | 21.5 | Black/tan; grizzle/tan |
| Alaskan malamute | WD | 66 | 61 | 38 | 34 | Light to dark grey and white markings |
| American cocker spaniel | GD | 38 | 35.5 | NS | NS | Almost any and particolour |
| Anatolian shepherd dog | WD | 79.5 | 79 | 60 | 59 | Fawn, black mask |
| Australian cattle dog | WD | 48 | 46 | <16 | <16 | Blue; speckled red |
| Australian silky terrier | TB | 25.5 | 25.5 | 4.5 | 4.5 | Blue or silver grey with tan markings on legs and face |
| Australian terrier | TER | 25.5 | 25.5 | 6 | 6 | Red grizzle or blue/tan |
| Basenji | H | 43 | 40.5 | 11 | 9.5 | Red; black; black/tan and white makings |
| Basset hound | H | 35.5 | 33 | 22.5 | 19.5 | Tricolour; any hound colour |
| Beagle | H | 40.5 | 33 | 9 | 9 | Tricolour; any hound colour |
| Bearded collie | WD | 56 | 51 | 22.5 | 20.5 | Black; grey; red/fawn; brown; sandy and white |
| Bedlington terrier | TER | 40.5 | 38 | 9 | 9 | Blue; blue/tan; liver; liver/tan; sandy |
| Belgian shepherd dogs: | | | | | | |
|   Groenendael | WD | 63.5 | 58.5 | NS | NS | Black |
|   Laekenois | WD | 63.5 | 58.5 | NS | NS | Rough coat, red/fawn |
|   Malinois | WD | 63.5 | 58.5 | NS | NS | Fawn with black overlay |
|   Tervueren | WD | 63.5 | 58.5 | NS | NS | Longcoat, fawn |

*continued on p. 130*

| Breed | Class | Average height at shoulder (cm) | | Average weight of adult (kg) | | Colour/markings |
|---|---|---|---|---|---|---|
| | | Male | Female | Male | Female | |
| Bernese mountain dog | WD | 66 | 61 | NS | NS | Black/tan and white markings |
| Bichon frise | TB | 28 | 28 | NS | NS | White |
| Bloodhound | H | 66 | 61 | 41 | 36.5 | Black/tan; red/tan; tawny |
| Border collie | WD | 53.5 | 51 | 23.5 | 19 | Variety permissible |
| Border terrier | TER | 30.5 | 28 | 6.5 | 5.5 | Red; wheaten; grizzle/tan; blue/tan |
| Borzoi | H | 73.5+ | 68.5+ | 41 | 34 | Any |
| Boston terrier | UB | NS | NS | 8 | 8 | Brindle/white; black/white |
| Bouvier des Flandres | WD | 66 | 61 | 38 | 34 | Fawn or grey shaded or black |
| Boxer | WD | 61 | 53.5 | 30 | 27 | Brindle; red; fawn and white markings |
| Briard | WD | 63.5 | 61 | 38.5 | 34 | Any solid colour |
| Brittany | GD | 50 | 48 | 15 | 13 | Orange/white; liver/white; black/white |
| Bull terrier | TER | 30.5 | 30.5 | 20.5 | 20.5 | White and head markings; brindle/white; black/white |
| Bull terrier (miniature) | TER | <35.5 | <35.5 | NS | NS | White; black/brindle; red; fawn; triclour |
| Bulldog | UB | NS | NS | 25 | 22.5 | Any except black; black/tan; Yellow |
| Bullmastiff | WD | 66 | 61 | 54.5 | 45.5 | Red; fawn; brindle and dark mask |
| Cairn terrier | TER | 25.5 | 24 | 6.5 | 6.5 | Red; wheaten; fawn; brindle |
| Canaan dog | UB | 56 | 56 | 23 | 23 | White; fawn; red; brown and white markings. Grey or black/tan not permitted. |
| Cavalier King Charles spaniel | TB | 32 | 32 | 7 | 7 | Black/tan; ruby; blenheim (chestnut and white); tricolour (black/white and tan markings) |
| Chesapeake Bay retriever | GD | 63.5 | 58.5 | 31 | 28 | Pale to dark brown |
| Chihuahua: | | | | | | |
|    Long coat | TB | NS | NS | 2 | 2 | Any |
|    Short coat | TB | NS | NS | 2 | 2 | Any |
| Chinese crested dog | TB | 30.5 | 28 | NS | NS | Any, plain or spotted |

| Breed | Class | Average height at shoulder (cm) | | Average weight of adult (kg) | | Colour/markings |
|---|---|---|---|---|---|---|
| | | Male | Female | Male | Female | |
| Chow chow | UB | 48.5 | 48.5 | 27 | 25 | Red; blue; black; fawn; cream |
| Clumber spaniel | GD | 45.5 | 45.5 | 28.5 | 24 | White and lemon markings |
| Cocker spaniel | GD | 40.5 | 38 | 13.5 | 13.5 | Black; red; gold; liver/white; tricolour; particolour |
| Collie (rough) | WD | 58.5 | 53.5 | 25 | 21.5 | Sable/white; tricolour; blue merle |
| Collie (smooth) | WD | 58.5 | 53.5 | 27 | 22.5 | Sable/white; tricolour; blue merle |
| Curly-coated retriever | GD | 68.5 | 63.5 | 34 | 34 | Liver or black |
| Dachshund (miniature) | H | NS | NS | <5 | <5 | Any except white |
| Dachshund (standard) | H | NS | NS | 9 | 9 | Any except white (long/smooth/wire-haired) |
| Dalmatian | UB | 61 | 56 | 27 | 25 | Black/white; liver/white |
| Dandie dinmont terrier | TER | 28 | 20.5 | 8 | 8 | Mustard; pepper |
| Deerhound | H | 76 | 71 | 45.5 | 36.5 | Shades of grey; yellow/fawn |
| Dobermann | WD | 68.5 | 65 | 37.5 | 33 | Black/rust; brown/rust; blue/rust |
| Elkhound | H | 52 | 49.5 | 22.5 | 19.5 | Grey |
| English setter | GD | 66 | 63.5 | 28.5 | 27 | Black/white; liver/white; lemon/white; tricolour |
| English springer spaniel | GD | 51 | 51 | 21.5 | 19 | Liver/white; black/white |
| English toy terrier | TB | <30.5 | <30.5 | <3.5 | <3.5 | Black/tan |
| Eskimo dog | WD | 63.5 | 58.5 | 45.5 | 41.5 | Any |
| Estrela mountain dog | WD | <76 | <76 | NS | NS | Any |
| Field spaniel | GD | <46 | <46 | 19 | 19 | Black; liver; roan |
| Finnish spitz | UB | 48.5 | 44.5 | 15 | 13.5 | Reddish brown; yellowish red |
| Flat-coated retriever | GD | NS | NS | 29.5 | 29.5 | Black or liver |
| Foxhound | H | 58.5 | 58.5 | 30.5 | 30.5 | Tan/white and black; tan/black and white; lemon/white pied; any hound colour |

*continued on p. 132*

| Breed | Class | Average height at shoulder (cm) | | Average weight of adult (kg) | | Colour/markings |
|---|---|---|---|---|---|---|
| | | Male | Female | Male | Female | |
| Fox terrier | TER | 39.5 | 39.5 | 8 | 7.5 | White and black or tan markings (smooth/wire-haired) |
| French bulldog | UB | NS | NS | 12.5 | 11 | Brindle fawn or pied |
| German shepherd dog (Alsatian) | WD | 63.5 | 58.5 | 36.5 | 29.5 | Any except white |
| German short-haired pointer | GD | 63.5 | 58.5 | 28.5 | 24 | Liver; liver and white spotted or ticked |
| German spitz: | | | | | | |
| Klein | UB | 25.5 | 25.5 | 3.5 | 3.5 | Orange/red, grey |
| Mittel | UB | 32 | 32 | NS | NS | Any |
| Glen of Imaal terrier | TER | 35.5 | 35.5 | 16 | 16 | Blue brindle or wheaten |
| Golden retriever | GD | 58.5 | 53.5 | 34 | 29.5 | Gold; cream |
| Gordon setter | GD | 66 | 62 | 29.5 | 25.5 | Black/chestnut |
| Great Dane | WD | 76+ | 71+ | 54.5 | 45.5 | Black; blue; white; red; fawn; brindle; particolour |
| Greyhound | H | 73.5 | 70 | 36.5 | 29.5 | Black; blue; white; red; fawn; brindle; particolour |
| Griffon Bruxellois | TB | NS | NS | 3.5 | 3.5 | Red/black; black/tan; rough or smooth coated |
| Hamiltonstovare | H | 58.5 | 58.5 | NS | NS | Black/brown |
| Hovawart | WD | <68.5 | <68.5 | <41.5 | <41.5 | Black; black/tan; pale brown |
| Hungarian vizsla | GD | 61 | 56 | <30 | <30 | Red |
| Ibizan hound | H | 63.5 | 63.5 | NS | NS | White; chestnut; orange solid colour |
| Irish setter | GD | 63.5 | 63.5 | 30.5 | 26 | Rich chestnut |
| Irish setter (red & white) | GD | 66 | 61 | 29.5 | 25 | White and red patches and flecking |
| Irish terrier | TER | 48.5 | 45.5 | 12 | 11.5 | Harsh wiry coat should be whole colours. Bright red, red wheaten or yellow red |
| Irish water spaniel | GD | 56 | 56 | 27 | 24 | Liver |
| Irish wolfhound | H | 79+ | 71+ | 54.5 | 41 | Black; grey; brindle; fawn; red; white |

| Breed | Class | Average height at shoulder (cm) | | Average weight of adult (kg) | | Colour/markings |
|---|---|---|---|---|---|---|
| | | Male | Female | Male | Female | |
| Italian greyhound | TB | 25.5 | 25.5 | 3 | 3 | Fawn; black; blue; cream; white; black/fawn/white |
| Italian spinone | GD | 66 | 61 | 34 | 29 | White with orange or brown speckling or marking |
| Japanese Akita | UB | 68.5 | 63.5 | 50 | 50 | All colours |
| Japanese Chin | TB | <18 | <18 | NS | NS | Black/white; red/white |
| Japanese Shiba Inu | UB | 38 | 38 | NS | NS | Red; black/tan; brindle; white; sesame and pinto |
| Japanese Spitz | UB | 38 | 30.5 | NS | NS | Pure white |
| Keeshund | UB | 45.5 | 43 | 19.5 | 18 | Wolf or ash grey and cream legs, feet |
| Kerry blue terrier | TER | 48.5 | 45.5 | 16 | 16 | Any shade of blue |
| King Charles spaniel | TB | 25.5 | 20.5 | 5 | 5 | Black/tan; tricolour; chestnut red and white |
| Komondor | WD | 66+ | 58.5+ | 61 | 50 | White corded coat |
| Labrador retriever | GD | 56 | 56 | 30.5 | 28.5 | Black; yellow; chocolate |
| Lakeland terrier | TER | <37 | <37 | 7.5 | 7 | Blue; blue/tan; black; black/tan; red; wheaten; grizzle |
| Lancashire heeler | WD | 30.5 | 25.5 | 6.5 | 6.5 | Black/tan markings |
| Large Munsterlander | GD | 61 | 58.5 | 27 | 29.5 | Black head, body white patched and flecked |
| Leonberger | UB | 76 | 71 | NS | NS | Light yellow; golden; red/brown with black |
| Lhaso Apso | UB | 25.5 | 23 | NS | NS | Gold; sandy; honey; grizzle; slate; smoke; particolours |
| Lowchen | TB | 30.5 | 30.5 | 3 | 3 | Any |
| Maltese | TB | 25.5 | 25.5 | NS | NS | Pure white |
| Manchester terrier | TER | 40.5 | 40.5 | <8 | <7.5 | Black and tan |
| Maremma sheepdog | WD | 71 | 66 | 43.5 | 38 | White |
| Mastiff | WD | NS | NS | 68 | 57 | Apricot; silver fawn; dark fawn brindle; black points |

*continued on p. 134*

| Breed | Class | Average height at shoulder (cm) | | Average weight of adult (kg) | | Colour/markings |
|---|---|---|---|---|---|---|
| | | Male | Female | Male | Female | |
| Miniature pinscher | TB | 30.5 | 25.5 | 3.5 | 3.5 | Red and black/tan |
| Neopolitan mastiff | WD | <72.5 | <68.5 | <68 | <68 | Black/grey |
| Newfoundland | WD | 71 | 66 | 66 | 52 | Dull black; brown; landseer (white/black) |
| Norfolk terrier | TER | 25.5 | 25.5 | 6.5 | 6.5 | Red; red/wheaten; black/tan; grizzle |
| Norwegian Buhund | WD | 43 | 43 | NS | NS | Wheaten; black/red; sable |
| Norwich terrier | TER | 28 | 25.5 | 6.5 | 6.5 | Red; wheaten; black/tan; grizzle |
| Old English sheepdog | WD | 61 | 56 | 36.5 | 29.5 | Grey; grizzle; blue; blue merle and white |
| Otterhound | H | <68.5 | <61 | 52 | 45.5 | Any |
| Papillon | TB | 28 | 20.5 | 2 | 2.5 | White and patches any colour except liver |
| Parson Jack Russell terrier | TER | 35.5 | 35.5 | NS | NS | White and coloured markings |
| Pekingese | TB | 18 | 18 | <5 | <5.5 | Any except liver |
| Petit basset griffon vendeen | H | 38 | 35.5 | 19 | 18 | Many colours |
| Petit bleu de Gascoine | H | 56 | 51 | NS | NS | Black markings on a white coat with black mottling |
| Pharoah hound | H | 61 | 58.5 | NS | NS | Tan |
| Pointer | GD | 66 | 63.5 | 29.5 | 25 | White and liver; black or lemon markings; whole black |
| Polish lowland sheepdog | WD | 51 | 51 | 19.5 | 18 | All colours; piebald |
| Pomeranian | TB | NS | NS | 2 | 2.5 | Red; orange; orange/sable; wolf/sable; beaver; blue; white; brown; chocolate; black |
| Poodle (miniature) | UB | <38 | <38 | 6 | 6 | Any solid colour |
| Poodle (standard) | UB | 38+ | 38+ | 34 | 29.5 | Any solid colour |
| Poodle (toy) | UB | <28 | <28 | 4.5 | 4.5 | Any solid colour |
| Portuguese water dog | WD | 56 | 51 | 25 | 23 | Black/white; brown/white |

| Breed | Class | Average height at shoulder (cm) | | Average weight of adult (kg) | | Colour/markings |
|---|---|---|---|---|---|---|
| | | Male | Female | Male | Female | |
| Pug | TB | NS | NS | 7.5 | 7.5 | Silver/fawn; apricot/fawn; black |
| Puli | WD | 43 | 43 | NS | NS | Black; white; rusty black; grey |
| Pyrenean mountain dog | WD | 71 | 66 | 50 | 41 | White; white and badger, grey or tan markings |
| Rhodesian ridgeback | H | 63.5 | 61 | 36.5 | 32 | Light red wheaten |
| Rottweiler | WD | 68.5 | 58.5 | 50 | 38.5 | Black/mahogany; black/tan |
| Saint Bernard | WD | <91.5 | <91.5 | 75 | 68 | Orange; mahogany/brindle; red brindle and white |
| Saluki | H | 65 | 57 | 24 | 19.5 | White; cream; gold; red fawn; black/tan; grizzle; tricolour |
| Samoyed | WD | 56 | 51 | 23 | 18 | White; white and biscuit; cream |
| Schipperke | UB | NS | NS | <8 | <8 | Black and other colours in UK |
| Schnauzer (giant) | WD | 66 | 61 | 45.5 | 41 | Pepper and salt; black |
| Schnauzer (miniature) | UB | 35.5 | 33 | 9 | 7.5 | Pepper and salt; black |
| Schnauzer (standard) | UB | 48.5 | 45.5 | 18 | 16 | Pepper and salt; black |
| Scottish terrier | TER | 28 | 25.5 | 9.5 | 9.5 | Black; brindle; wheaten |
| Sealyham terrier | TER | 30.5 | 25.5 | <9 | <8 | White and badger, brown or lemon markings |
| Shar-pei | UB | <51 | <51 | <23 | <23 | Black; red; fawn; cream |
| Shetland sheepdog | WD | 37 | 35.5 | 9 | 9 | Black/tan; black/white; tricolour; sable/white; blue merle and white |
| Shih Tzu | UB | <26.5 | <26.5 | 7 | 7 | Any |
| Siberian husky | WD | 58.5 | 53.5 | 26 | 20.5 | All colours |
| Skye terrier | TER | 25.5 | 25.5 | 11.5 | 10 | Grey, fawn, cream and black |
| Soft-coated wheaten terrier | TER | 45.5 | 45.5 | 18 | 18 | Fawn/gold |
| Staffordshire bull terrier | TER | 40.5 | 35.5 | 15 | 13 | Black; blue; red; brindle; fawn and white; white |
| Sussex spaniel | GD | 40.5 | 38 | 20.5 | 18 | Rich golden liver |
| Swedish Vallhund | WD | 33 | 30.5 | 8 | 12.5 | Grey shaded; red shaded |

*continued on p. 136*

| Breed | Class | Average height at shoulder (cm) | | Average weight of adult (kg) | | Colour/markings |
|---|---|---|---|---|---|---|
| | | Male | Female | Male | Female | |
| Tibetan mastiff | WD | 66 | 61 | NS | NS | Rich black; tan; brown; shades of gold/grey |
| Tibetan spaniel | UB | 25.5 | 25.5 | 5.5 | 5.5 | Any except chocolate or liver |
| Tibetan terrier | UB | 38 | 35.5 | 12 | 12 | White; cream; grey; gold; particolour; black |
| Weimaraner | GD | 63.5 | 61 | 27 | 22.5 | Silver; mouse/grey |
| Welsh corgi (Cardigan) | WD | 30.5 | 30.5 | 11 | 10 | Any except pure white |
| Welsh corgi (Pembroke) | WD | 30.5 | 25.5 | 10 | 9 | Red; sable; fawn; black/tan and white |
| Welsh springer spaniel | GD | 45.5 | 45.5 | 17 | 17 | Red and white |
| Welsh terrier | TER | <39.5 | <39.5 | 9.5 | 9 | Black/tan; grizzle/tan |
| West highland white terrier | TER | 28 | 28 | 8.5 | 7.5 | White |
| Whippet | H | 48.5 | 45.5 | 11.5 | 10 | Any |
| Yorkshire terrier | TB | 20.5 | 18 | <3 | <3 | Steel blue/tan |

# Appendix 2: Dog and Cat Diets

Hill's Pet Products Ltd.
1 The Beacons
Beaconsfield Road
Hatfield
Hertfordshire
AL10 8EQ

Tel: 0707 276660

An alphabetical list of some of the manufacturers of dog and cat diets, giving details of their name, address, telephone number and details of the products which they sell.

| Product | Reference | Indications | Canned (g) | Dry (kg) |
|---------|-----------|-------------|------------|----------|
| *Canine* | | | | |
| c/d | Calculi | An aid in preventing re-occurrence of struvite calculi; adult maintenance | 447 | 5<br>10 |
| d/d | Dermatological | Dermatitis or gastroenteritis associated with food allergy; as a dietary trial for above | 447 | 5 |
| g/d | Geriatric | The geriatric dog; endocrine imbalance; early renal and congestive heart disease | 447 | 5 |
| h/d | Heart | Sodium and fluid retention in advanced congestive heart failure; sodium retention or hypertension in renal and liver disease | 447 | 5 |
| i/d | Intestinal | Gastro-intestinal disease (vomiting, diarrhoea); postgastro-intestinal surgery; liver disease; pancreatic insufficiency; early weaning; bloat | 447 | 5<br>10 |
| k/d | Kidney | Acute and chronic renal failure; liver disease; early congestive heart failure | 447 | 5 |
| p/d | Protein | Debilitation; malnutrition and deficiency diseases; skeletal disease and fractures; reproduction and growth | 447 | 5 |
| r/d | Reducing | Obesity in adult dogs; fibre-responsive diseases in overweight animals, e.g. diabetes mellitus, constipation, lymphangiectasia and colitis | 425 | 5<br>10 |
| s/d | Struvite | Dissolution of struvite calculi in conjunction with medical therapy | 447 | |
| u/d | Uraemia/urolithiasis | Advanced renal failure; advanced liver disease and management of urate, cystine, oxalate urolithiasis; copper storage disease | 447 | 5 |
| w/d | Weight control | Management of fibre-responsive diseases in normal weight animals (see r/d); maintenance of weight loss in the previously obese dog | 447 | 5 |
| *Feline* | | | | |
| c/d | Calculi/cystitis | An aid in the management of FLUTD; adult maintenance; anorexia – cat and dog; gastro-intestinal conditions | 425 | 2<br>5 |

Column heading above Canned (g) and Dry (kg): **Packaging**

*continued on p. 138*

| Product | Reference | Indications | Packaging | |
|---------|-----------|-------------|-----------|---|
| | | | Canned (g) | Dry (kg) |
| d/d | Dermatological | Dermatitis or gastroenteritis associated with food allergy; as a dietary trial for above | 425 | |
| h/d | Heart | Congestive heart failure; hepatic disease; oedema; ascites; hypertension | 425 | |
| k/d | Kidney | Renal disease; liver disease; management of oxalate urolithiasis | 425 | 5 |
| p/d | Protein | Malnutrition; debilitation and deficiency diseases; skeletal disease and fractures; pregnancy/lactation; growth | 425 | 5 |
| r/d | Reducing | Obesity in adult cats; fibre-responsive diseases, such as constipation, hair-balls and diabetes mellitus in overweight animals | 425 | 5 |
| s/d | Struvite | Dissolution of struvite calculi in urolithiasis, and crystals in feline urological syndrome, in conjunction with medical therapy | 425 | 5 |
| w/d | Weight control | Management of fibre-responsive diseases in normal weight animals (see r/d); maintenance of weight loss in the previously obese cat | 425 | 2 |

Leander International Pet Foods Ltd.
Arden Grange
London Road
Albourne
Hassocks
Sussex
BN6 9BJ

Tel: 0273 833390

| Product | Characteristics | Ingredients |
| --- | --- | --- |
| *Canine* | [Available in 200 g (trial size), 1 kg, 3 kg, 7.5 kg and 15 kg bags] | |
| Eukanuba Premium | Provides optimum nutrition through all stages of a dog's life. It is an ideal food for all dogs with a normal to high energy requirement, and also working dogs, pregnant or lactating bitches and recuperating animals. It has been found to be very helpful in the management of a number of conditions including colitis and skin complaints | Chicken meal, ground corn, chicken, rice flour, chicken fat, beet pulp, dried whole egg, brewer's dried yeast, vitamins, minerals and trace elements |
| Eukanuba Regular | Provides an excellent maintenance diet for the adult dog with a normal level of activity | Chicken meal, ground corn, rice flour, animal fat, beet pulp, dried whole egg, brewer's dried yeast, vitamins, minerals and trace elements |
| Eukanuba Light | A calorie-reduced diet which does not sacrifice nutritional value. It is designed for the adult dog with a below average activity level, or for those with a tendency to be overweight | Ground corn, chicken meal, rice flour, chicken fat, beet pulp, dried whole egg, fish meal, brewer's dried yeast, chicken liver meal, vitamins, minerals and trace elements |
| Eukanuba Junior | Designed to meet the optimum nutritional needs of the older puppy. It is an excellent diet for puppies from the larger and giant breeds where it is essential to control growth rate | Chicken meal, ground corn, rice flour, chicken fat, animal fat, beet pulp, dried whole egg, brewer's dried yeast, chicken liver meal, vitamins, minerals and trace elements |
| Eukanuba Puppy | Designed to meet the optimum nutritional needs of the growing puppy. It is an excellent weaning food | Chicken meal, ground corn, rice flour, chicken fat, beet pulp, animal fat, dried whole egg, brewer's dried yeast, vitamins, minerals and trace elements |
| *Feline* Dried foods | [Available in 200 g (sample size), 1 kg, 3 kg, 7.5 kg and 15 kg bags] | |
| IAMS Cat Food | Formulated to provide the optimum nutritional needs for all stages of the cat's life. It is also suitable for both pregnant and lactating queens. It has a magnesium level <0.076 mg/kg and is high in meat protein which helps produce an acid urine, reducing the risk of FLUTD. It is high in natural | Chicken meal, chicken, rice flour, ground corn, poultry fat, dried whole egg, beet pulp, fish meal, brewer's dried yeast, chicken liver meal, poultry fat, fish meal, vitamins, and trace elements |

*continued on p. 140*

| Product | Characteristics | Ingredients |
|---------|-----------------|-------------|
| IAMS Cat Food *contd* | taurine and under controlled studies produced an average plasma taurine level of 105 nmol/ml | |
| IAMS Kitten Food | Formulated to provide the optimum nutritional needs for growing kittens, suitable to wean kittens onto from 3 weeks of age | Chicken meal, chicken, rice flour, ground corn, poultry fat, dried whole egg, beet pulp, fish meal, brewer's dried yeast, chicken liver meal, vitamins and trace elements |
| Canned foods | [Based on fresh chicken, ocean fish and fresh liver and beef; low in magnesium and high in animal protein, producing an acidic urine which reduces the risk of feline urological syndrome (available in 170 g cans)] | |
| IAMS Ocean Fish Formula | | Mackerel, liver, poultry fat, dried whole egg, rice flour, vitamins, minerals and trace elements |
| IAMS Chicken Formula | | Chicken, poultry liver, dried whole egg, rice flour, vitamins, minerals and trace elements |
| IAMS Beef and Liver Formula | | Beef liver, beef, dried whole egg, rice flour, poultry fat, vitamins, minerals and trace elements |

Veterinary considerations
The IAMS foods have proved to be of practical benefit in the management of diseases where dietary allergy is considered to be a contributing factor, cats that are predisposed to FLUTD, animals where faecal output needs to be minimal, and animals with poor skin and coat condition.

Pedigree Petfoods
Veterinary Services
Waltham on the Wolds
Melton Mowbray
Leicestershire
LE14 4RS

Tel: 0664 410000

| Product | Characteristics | Indications | Contraindications | Packaging Canned (g) | Dry (kg) |
|---|---|---|---|---|---|
| *Canine* Low-calorie diet | Low energy density; increased levels of vitamins and minerals; highly palatable | Obesity/overweight | Growing puppies; pregnant/lactating bitches; working dogs | 400 | – |
| Calorie-control diet | Low energy density; increased levels of vitamins and minerals; highly palatable | Obesity/overweight | Growing puppies; pregnant/lactating bitches; working dogs | – | 3 |
| Low-fat diet | Restricted fat content; highly palatable, easily digestible | Acute/chronic diarrhoea | None | 400 | 4 |
| Selected protein diet | Protein content derived solely from chicken and rice; no gluten or dairy products; highly palatable, easily digestible | Acute/chronic diarrhoea; dietary intolerance or hypersensitivity | None | 400 | – |
| Low-protein diet | Reduced level of protein; energy content derived mainly from non-protein sources; increased levels of B vitamins; restricted phosphorus, no added sodium; highly palatable, easily digestible | Chronic kidney failure | Growing puppies; pregnant/lactating bitches; dogs with severe proteinuria | 400 | 4 |
| Medium protein diet | Reduced level of protein; energy content derived mainly from non-protein sources; increased levels of B vitamins; restricted phosphorus, no added sodium; highly palatable, easily digestible | Reduced kidney function (e.g. geriatric dogs) | Growing puppies; pregnant/lactating bitches; dogs with severe proteinuria | 400 | – |
| Low-sodium diet | Restricted sodium; high BV protein; increased level of potassium; increased levels of B vitamins; highly palatable, easily digestible | Congestive heart failure/hypertension | Growing puppies; pregnant/lactating bitches | 400 | – |

*continued on p. 142*

| Product | Characteristics | Indications | Contraindications | Packaging Canned (g) | Dry (kg) |
|---------|----------------|-------------|-------------------|----------------------|----------|
| Concentration diet | Concentrated and balanced source of nutrients; highly palatable, easily digestible | Convalescence; pregnancy/lactation; growth | None | 400 | – |
| Conditioning diet | High quality protein; nutritionally balanced; highly palatable, easily digestible | Adult maintenance | None | 400 | 4 |
| *Feline* Low-calorie diet | Low energy density; increased levels of vitamins and minerals; highly palatable | Obesity/overweight | Growing kittens; pregnant/lactating queens | 200 | – |
| Selected protein diet | Protein content derived solely from chicken and rice; no gluten or dairy products; highly palatable, easily digestible | Acute/chronic diarrhoea; dietary intolerance or hypersensitivity | None | 200 | – |
| Low-protein diet | Reduced level of protein; energy content derived mainly from non-protein sources; increased levels of B vitamins; increased level of potassium; restricted phosphorus, no added sodium; highly palatable, easily digestible | Chronic kidney failure | Growing kittens; pregnant/lactating queens; cats with severe proteinuria | 200 | – |
| pH control diet | Low magnesium content; produces an acidic urine; increased levels of taurine and potassium; highly palatable, easily digestible | FLUTD | Growing kittens; pregnant/lactating queens; cats receiving urinary acidifiers | 200 | – |
| Concentration diet | Concentrated and balanced source of nutrients; highly palatable, easily digestible | Convalescence; pregnancy/lactation; growth | None | 200 | – |
| Conditioning diet | High quality protein; nutritionally balanced; highly palatable, easily digestible | Adult maintenance | None | 200 | – |

Wafcol
The Nutrition Bakery
Haigh Avenue
Stockport
SK4 1NU

Tel: 061 480 2781

| Product | Characteristics | Indications |
|---|---|---|
| *Canine* | | |
| Rite-weight | Lower calorie diet | Obesity; weight control; diabetes mellitus |
| Veteran | Lower protein diet | CRF; incontinence; gastric dilation; ageing dogs; digestive disorders |
| *Hypoallergenic diets* | | |
| Special '21' | Free of gluten, red meat and dairy products | Colitis; allergic dermatoses; hyperactivity; gluten intolerance; pancreatic insufficiency |
| Vegetarian | Free of all meat products | Colitis; diarrhoea; allergic dermatoses; aggression; hyperactivity; anal sac impaction; constipation; diabetes mellitus |
| '20' | Free of maize | Maize intolerance; allergic dermatoses; anal sac impaction; diarrhoea |

# Glossary

The following is a glossary of terms which are either used in this volume or are relevant to further reading in related fields of nutrition and clinical nutrition.

**Absorption** The process of uptake of a nutrient or other ingested substance from the gastro-intestinal tract by the outermost cells of the walls of the tract.

**Ad libitum feeding** The system in which the food supply is unrestricted at all times (in contrast to meal feeding).

**Allowance** The amount of a nutrient which is given under practical conditions to meet the daily requirement of the animal. A margin of safety is included to allow for factors which cannot be readily quantified.

**Anabolism** The process of synthesis of complex organic molecules from simpler ones in the tissues.

**Anorexia** Lack or loss of appetite.

**Apparent digestibility** The amount of a nutrient ingested minus the amount voided in the faeces (including any of endogenous origin) during a period of time, expressed as a proportion of the amount ingested.

$$\text{Apparent digestibility} = \frac{\text{amount ingested} - \text{amount in faeces}}{\text{amount ingested}}$$

**Ascites** Effusion and accumulation of serous fluid in the abdominal cavity.

**Availability** The proportion of a nutrient supplied in the food which, at a stated rate of inclusion and level of feeding, can be absorbed and utilized by the animal to meet its net requirement.

**Azotaemia** Excess of urea or other nitrogenous compounds in the blood.

**Basal metabolic rate (BMR)** The amount of energy required to maintain the activity of the internal organs and the body temperature while the animal is at rest and fasting. Since heat loss and other metabolic functions are more closely related to surface area than to body weight, basal energy expenditure (kcal) is usually expressed as a function of surface area or $W(\text{kg})^{0.75}$.

**b.i.d.** Twice a day (*bis in die*).

**Biological value (BV)** The proportion of a food protein which can be utilized by an animal for synthesizing body tissues and compounds. Using total nitrogen (N) as a measure of protein, the biological value (BV) is obtained by measuring N intake and output in urine and faeces.

$$BV = \frac{\text{N intake} - (\text{faecal}\star \text{ N} + \text{urinary}\star \text{ N})}{\text{N intake} - \text{faecal}\star \text{ N}}$$

$\star$After deduction of endogenous or obligatory faecal or urinary N. Thus, the theoretical maximum BV of 1 would be attained if net urinary N excretion were 0. If corrections are not made for endogenous excretory losses, the value obtained is the *apparent biological value (ABV)*.

**Calorie (cal)** A measure of energy (the amount of heat required to raise the temperature of 1 g of water by 1°C). The approximate energy available to the animal from its food can be obtained by multiplying the protein, fat and carbohydrate concentration (%) by factors: protein $\times$ 3.5, fat $\times$ 8.46 and carbohydrate $\times$ 3.5, the result being expressed as kilocalories (kcal) of metabolizable energy (ME)/100 g of food. Estimates of ME values are substantially affected by the digestibility of the food. 4.184 joules (J) are equivalent to 1 cal.

**Catabolism** The process of breaking down complex molecules to simpler ones in the tissues.

**Cirrhosis** Liver disease characterized by loss of lobular structure with fibrosis and nodular regeneration.

**Critical temperature** The lower critical temperature is the environmental temperature below which the body's normal rate of heat production is insufficient to compensate for heat loss. Heat production and thus energy requirement increases below this point in order to maintain body temperature. If the environmental temperature drops below this capacity to increase heat production, the body cools (hypothermia) and metabolic rate decreases. The upper critical temperature is when heat loss to the environment by passive means can no longer dissipate the heat produced by normal metabolism. Active heat-dissipating mechanisms such as sweating or panting are necessary to prevent body temperature rising above normal. Further increases in environmental temperature may exceed the capacity of these active mechanisms and body temperature increases (hyperthermia).

**Digestible energy (DE)** The gross energy (GE) (or heat of combustion) of the food minus the GE of the corresponding faeces expressed as kcal or kJ/g of food. Usually DE = 0.75–0.80 GE.

**Digestion** The process of converting food in the alimentary tract into substances which can be absorbed through the wall of the tract.

**DM** Dry matter.

**Dyschesia** Difficult or painful evacuation of faeces from the rectum.

**Endocrine** Secreting inwardly (hormone) into the blood.

**Endogenous loss** The amount of a nutrient which originates from the tissues of the animal and is excreted in the faeces or urine or both.

**Essential amino acids** Those amino acids which are not synthesized in the tissues of the animal in amounts sufficient to meet its requirements and must therefore be supplied in the food.

**Exocrine** Secreting outwardly via a duct.

**Gross energy (GE)** The heat of combustion of a unit weight of material (food, excreta) as determined by burning it in a bomb calorimeter.

**Haematochesia** Passage of bloody stools.

**Hyper-** A prefix meaning above, beyond, more than normal, excessive; e.g. hypercalcaemia, an excess of calcium in the blood; hyperemesis, excesssive vomiting; hypervitaminosis, a condition due to the ingestion of excessive amounts of one or more vitamins; hyperventilation, an abnormal increase in the rate and/or depth of breathing.

**Hypo-** A prefix signifying beneath, under, below normal, deficient, e.g. hypocalcaemia, a blood calcium concentration below normal, etc.

**Icterus** Jaundice.

**IV** Intravenous.

**Joule (J)** SI unit of energy. 4.184 J = 1 cal, $10^3$ joules = 1 kJ, $10^6$ joules = 1 MJ.

**Lymphangiectasia** Dilatation of the lymphatic vessels.

**Meal feeding** A system of feeding whereby the food is provided on one or more occasions during the day in amounts which the animal will consume more or less completely on that or those occasions.

**Metabolism** Term embracing anabolism and catabolism.

**Metabolizable energy (ME)** The digestible energy (DE) of unit weight of food minus the heat of combustion of the corresponding urine. ME $\approx$ 0.96 DE.

**Nitrogen retention (NR)** A measure of the proportion of protein (N $\times$ 6.25) in the food which is retained by the animal. NR = N in the food − (Faecal N + urinary N).

**Obligatory loss** The amount of a nutrient that has undergone metabolic change in the animal body and which is unavoidably excreted in the urine or faeces or both, irrespective of the presence or absence of the nutrient in the diet.

**o.d.** Once a day (*omni die*).

**Pathognomonic** Specifically distinctive or characteristic of a disease or pathologic condition.

**Polydipsia** Excessive thirst.

**Polyuria** Passage of increased volumes of urine.

**Portosystemic shunt** An abnormal short-circuit of blood from portal to systemic circulation, thus bypassing the liver.

**Protein (crude)** Estimated protein content from chemically determined nitrogen content (usually defined as N $\times$ 6.25). May significantly overestimate protein content if non-protein N is present.

**Protein-sparing effect** Sparing the oxidation of protein as an energy source by providing additional carbohydrate and/or fat.

**Ptyalism** Excessive flow of saliva.

**Requirement** The amount of a nutrient which must be supplied in the diet to meet the Requirement (net).

**Requirement (net)** The quantity of a nutrient which should be absorbed by a normal healthy animal in order to meet its needs for maintenance and, if stated, for growth or for reproduction.

**Steatorrhoea** Excessive amount of fat in the faeces.

**Tenesmus** Straining to pass faeces or urine.

**t.i.d.** Three times a day (*ter in die*).

**True digestibility (TD)** The proportion of a nutrient which has been ingested (in the food) and absorbed, expressed as a decimal of nutrient ingested:

$$TD = \frac{\text{Amount ingested} - (\text{amount in faeces} - \text{endogenous faecal loss})}{\text{amount ingested}}$$

**Vitamins** A general term for a number of unrelated organic substances which occur in many foods in small amounts and are necessary in trace amounts for the normal functioning of the body. They may be water- or fat-soluble.

# Index